# Public Health Mini-Guide
# **Obesity**

**Nick Townsend**
Senior Researcher, University of Oxford, Oxford, UK

**Angela Scriven**
Reader in Health Promotion, Brunel University, London, UK

Series editor:
**Angela Scriven**

CHURCHILL
LIVINGSTONE

ELSEVIER    Edinburgh   London   New York   Oxford   Philadelphia   St Louis   Sydney   Toronto   2014

# CHURCHILL
# LIVINGSTONE
### ELSEVIER

© 2014 Elsevier Ltd. All rights reserved.

ISBN 9780702046346

**British Library Cataloguing in Publication Data**
A catalogue record for this book is available from the British Library

**Library of Congress Cataloging in Publication Data**
A catalog record for this book is available from the Library of Congress

**Notices**
Knowledge and best practice in this field are constantly changing. As new research and experience broaden our understanding, changes in research methods, professional practices, or medical treatment may become necessary.

Practitioners and researchers must always rely on their own experience and knowledge in evaluating and using any information, methods, compounds, or experiments described herein. In using such information or methods they should be mindful of their own safety and the safety of others, including parties for whom they have a professional responsibility.

With respect to any drug or pharmaceutical products identified, readers are advised to check the most current information provided (i) on procedures featured or (ii) by the manufacturer of each product to be administered, to verify the recommended dose or formula, the method and duration of administration, and contraindications. It is the responsibility of practitioners, relying on their own experience and knowledge of their patients, to make diagnoses, to determine dosages and the best treatment for each individual patient, and to take all appropriate safety precautions.

To the fullest extent of the law, neither the Publisher nor the authors, contributors, or editors, assume any liability for any injury and/or damage to persons or property as a matter of products liability, negligence or otherwise, or from any use or operation of any methods, products, instructions, or ideas contained in the material herein.

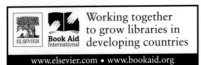
Printed in China

# Contents

*Titles in the* Public Health Mini-Guide *series*:

*Obesity*
Nick Townsend, Angela Scriven
ISBN 9780702046346

*Alcohol Misuse* (forthcoming)
Ken Barrie, Angela Scriven
ISBN 9780702046384

*Diabetes* (forthcoming)
Josie Evans, Angela Scriven
ISBN 9780702046377

# Series preface

The UK Government highlighted in the Foreword to its strategy for public health in England, the *Healthy Lives, Healthy People* White Paper[1] some of the public health challenges that are facing those working to improve public health: 'Britain is now the most obese nation in Europe. We have among the worst rates of sexually transmitted infections recorded, a relatively large population of problem drug users and rising levels of harm from alcohol. Smoking alone claims over 80,000 lives in every year. Experts estimate that tackling poor mental health could reduce our overall disease burden by nearly a quarter. Health inequalities between rich and poor have been getting progressively worse'.

The public health targets are clear both in the White Paper and in *Our Health and Wellbeing Today*,[2] published to accompany the White Paper, with the targets being supplemented by further policy drivers for mental health, tobacco control, obesity, sexual health and the wider determinants. The proposals and identified priorities in the White Paper apply to England, but they are of equal concern in the Devolved Administrations and globally, as evidenced in World Health Organization reports (www.who.int/whr/en/index.html). The *Public Health Mini-Guides* series covers some of the key health targets identified by the UK Government and WHO. The *Mini-Guides* highlight, in a concise, easily accessible manner, what the problems are and the range of potential solutions available to those professionals with a responsibility to promote health.

## What the *Public Health Mini-Guides* provide

The *Mini-Guides* are written to provide up-to-date, evidence-based information in a convenient pocket-sized format, on a range of current key public health topics. They will support the work of health and social care practitioners and students on courses related to public health and health promotion.

Each volume provides an objective and balanced introduction to an overview of the epidemiological, scientific, and other factors relating to public health. The *Mini-Guides* are structured to provide easy access to information. The first chapters cover background information needed to quickly understand the issue, including the epidemiology, demography and physiology. The later chapters examine examples of public health action to address the issue, covering health promotion intervention, legislative and other measures. The *Mini-Guides* are designed to be essential reference texts for students, practitioners and researchers with a professional interest in public health and health promotion.

Uxbridge, 2012                                                                 Angela Scriven

## References

1. The Stationery Office. Healthy Lives, Healthy People. White Paper. 2010.
2. Department of Health. Our Health and Wellbeing Today. London: Department of Health; 2010.

# Preface

Obesity and its linked morbidity and mortality place a burden not only on the individual but also on society as a whole. It is a significant public health challenge on a global scale. This *Mini Guide* presents key themes relating to this challenge, including the means of measuring obesity, the most recent prevalence and trends, and the health consequences and causes of obesity, along with approaches to counter obesity both at an individual and a population level.

Chapter 1 starts with defining obesity, and then critiques the various measures by assessing their strengths and weaknesses. Obesity in children and the use of growth charts is considered alongside the range of thresholds available (UK90, CDC, IOTF, WHO) and an explanation of the difficulties in using them. The chapter finishes with a short piece on the adiposity rebound and evidence of predicting future obesity. Chapter 2 covers prevalence and trends with regional, ethnic and social differences in prevalence in the UK compared to international data and estimated future trends. Chapter 3 examines the health consequences of obesity, highlighting any extra complications from obesity in childhood. Relative risks, where available, of some of these morbidities are presented. Causal pathways are discussed and the difficulty in separating obesity as a risk factor is explained alongside the evidence of obesity related mortality. Chapter 4 covers the causes of obesity and their interrelations and demonstrates the complex nature of the determination of obesity. Chapter 5 deals with ways of combating obesity at the individual level with description of how to treat obese individuals, from diet and exercise to medical intervention including NICE recommendations. Chapter 6 assesses how to intervene at a population rather than individual level, introducing a public health approach to preventing obesity, including policy impacts.

Each chapter covers important content on these themes with suggestions on where readers can find more information through links to webpages, resources and further reading. Understanding is facilitated through Case Studies, examples in Boxes, Thinking Points and an end-of-chapter set of Summary Points.

# 1 Defining the obesity problem

## What is obesity?

Obesity is a medical condition characterised by an excess of adipose tissue (fat) in the body that may have adverse effect on the health of an individual[1-4] (see Chapter 3 for detailed coverage of the health risks of obesity). The World Health Organization (WHO) similarly defines overweight and obesity as abnormal or excessive fat accumulation that presents a risk to health.[5] This is an important definition, as it indicates what to measure when investigating obesity.

## Measuring obesity

**Screening programmes** These are large-scale programmes that identify those who are at risk from obesity-related ill health. They should be accompanied by an explicit intention to prevent and also reduce the prevalence of obesity in the population.[6-9] For example, if a General Practice (GP) surgery is routinely measuring patients visiting their practice in order to identify those who are overweight or obese, it is important that when individuals are classified within high-risk weight status thresholds, they receive suitable treatment to enable them to reduce their weight in a healthy manner.

**Surveillance programmes** The aim here is to monitor the levels of obesity in a population rather than to identify those who require treatment.[9-11] Within surveillance programmes, data are usually anonymised, meaning that no routine feedback of individualised results is provided, nor is any formal link to treatment maintained. Data collected from these programmes enable the identification and monitoring of trends over time and assist in the targeting of interventions. Additionally, information from surveillance programmes may be used to analyse different causal and contributory factors for overweight and obesity, supporting the development of effective interventions and public health approaches to tackle obesity[12,13] (see Chapter 6 for an overview of public health obesity interventions).

On occasions programmes may straddle the line between screening and surveillance, such as the National Child Measurement Programme (NCMP) in England (see the NCMP Case Study in Box 1.1).

---

## ! Thinking points

1. Some people object to the collection of measurements related to obesity, although screening for other health conditions is welcomed; why is there this disparity?
2. What unintended harms can arise from running obesity measuring programmes?
3. Is it ethically sound to run a surveillance programme in which those identified as at risk of ill health are not informed?
4. With changes to the NHS in England, the running of the NCMP may have to change; should it be retained, and what should be saved in order to link future obesity measurement findings to earlier data?

---

### Box 1.1 Case study: National Child Measurement Programme

The National Child Measurement Programme (NCMP) for England was established in 2005/06. The NCMP collects population-level surveillance data for children through taking annual measurements of height and weight for Reception year (typically aged 4–5 years) and Year 6 (typically aged 10–11 years) primary school pupils.[14] The measurement exercise was coordinated locally by Primary Care Trusts (PCTs) with the support and cooperation of schools.[15] PCTs were freestanding statutory bodies of the National Health Service (NHS) that had the responsibility for securing the provision of a full range of primary care services for the local populations. There were 152 PCTs covering all of England within which the collection of NCMP data was coordinated. However, changes to the structure of the NHS under the Health and Social Care Bill 2011 announced the abolishment of PCTs by 2013, with the public health aspects of the PCTs taken on by local councils.[16] With the abolition of the PCTs, responsibility for NCMP measurement was taken on by Local Authorities with central collation of the data conducted by the Health and Social Care Information Centre (HSCIC) which was formally known as the NHS Information Centre. With the abolition of the PCTs in 2013 this measurement became the responsibility of Local Authorities. Authorities can undertake measurements at any time during the school year.[17] Height and weight measurements are taken by health professionals,

*Continued*

usually school nurses, in a room or screened area. Measurements are taken with children in 'normal light indoor clothing' without shoes or coats. The weight is recorded in kilograms (kg) to the first decimal place (the nearest 100 g) and height is recorded in cm to the first decimal place (the nearest mm).[17] Some differences between PCTs in the collection and recording of data had been found to influence prevalence estimates at the PCT level.[18]

The NCMP data are key to improving understanding of overweight and obesity in children. They are used at a national level to inform policy and locally to inform the planning and commissioning of services. The NCMP also provides local areas with an opportunity to raise public awareness of child obesity as well as informing parents of a child's result, sent through a letter.[14,19] In addition, the Public Health England Obesity Knowledge and Intelligence team (formerly the National Obesity Observatory) presents NCMP data in an e-Atlas – an interactive mapping tool that enables the user to compare a range of indicators, examine correlations and allows regional and national comparisons: www.noo.org.uk/visualisation/eatlas

Further details on the NCMP can be found at the Obesity Knowledge and Intelligence team website (www.noo.org.uk/NCMP) and through the Health and Social Care Information Service (http://www.hscic.gov.uk/ncmp).

## Measurement of obesity

There is a lot of evidence to suggest that self-reported height and weight data are unreliable[20–22] with indications that overweight or obese adults tend to underestimate their weight[20,22–24] or overestimate their height,[20,23] with the degree to which this is done varying by age;[21,23,25] sex;[20–22] and ethnicity.[26,27] Similar results have also been found with adolescents[28–32] and with parents reporting on the weight of their children.[33–35] It is imperative, therefore, in collecting data on obesity, or in assessing an individual's risk of obesity-related ill health, that objective accurate measures are taken.

There are a number of measures which can be taken to identify those at risk from obesity-related ill health. These range from the relatively simple Body Mass Index (BMI), which acts as a proxy for excess adiposity by providing a weight for height adjusted measure, to cross-sectional scans such as magnetic resonance imaging (MRI) and computerized tomography (CT), which provide an accurate measurement of amount and distribution of adipose tissue within an individual's body. In general the more complex measuring processes are the more time consuming and expensive to conduct, making it challenging to use them on a large scale.

### Common measures of obesity
#### Body Mass Index (BMI)

BMI is an index of weight-for-height that is most commonly used to classify weight status. It is calculated as weight in kilograms divided by the square of height in metres (Box 1.2).

**Box 1.2 Formula for Body Mass Index (BMI)**

$$BMI = \frac{weight\,(kilograms)}{height\,(metres)^2}$$

**Table 1.1** Classification of weight status in adults according to BMI

| BMI RANGE (kg/m²) | CLASSIFICATION |
|---|---|
| <18.5 | Underweight |
| 18.5–24.9 | Normal weight |
| 25–29.9 | Overweight |
| 30–39.9 | Obese |
| ≥40 | Morbidly obese |

Weight status is classified according to BMI from WHO classifications that are based largely on the association between BMI and mortality[36] (Table 1.1). These values are age-independent and the same for both sexes.

The National Institute for Health and Care Excellence (NICE) and the Australian Government National Health and Medical Research Council (NHMRC) in Australia recommend using BMI as a measure of overweight in adults, but both warn that this should be interpreted with caution as it does not provide a direct measure of adiposity.[37,38] The National Institutes for Health (NIH) in the United States published guidelines in 1998 that are still promoted by the Centers for Disease Control and Prevention (CDC) recommending the use of BMI as a practical approach in the clinical setting.[39]

***Weaknesses and strengths of BMI***
As BMI is an index of mass for height it cannot distinguish between weight associated with muscle mass and weight associated with fat mass. The relationship between BMI and adiposity can, therefore, vary according to the build of an individual. This means that an equal BMI might not correspond to the same degree of adiposity across populations, and it can be difficult to use BMI when comparing between subgroups of a population as this association may differ by sex,[40] age[41,42] and ethnic group.[43]

Additionally, although we have much evidence that increasing BMI is associated with increasing ill health,[44] the cut-offs used to classify overweight and obesity from BMI are statistical, as they are assigned to certain percentiles of the reference population,[45] rather than being truly health based. This means that the thresholds should not be used as an exact measure of risk. For example, individuals whose BMI lies either side of a threshold are more similar than those at opposing ends of a weight category. BMI is a continuous measure; therefore converting it to a discrete measures such as weight status reduces precision and variability and may also misrepresent trends on a population level as it can lead to disproportionate change.[46] It is possible, however, to avoid this by mapping changes in the population using smoothed curves of BMI, which provide a clearer description of what changes are occurring on a population level.

Despite concerns over BMI, it has consistently been found to be a reasonable proxy for body fat when used for large numbers of individuals. Research comparing BMI to body fat percentage as measured through accurate measurement of adiposity have found a strong correlation between BMI and total body fat,[47] as well as total abdominal adipose tissue,[48] although this correlation was not strong for visceral adipose tissue.[48] BMI is also closely correlated to obesity ill health on a population level and is a non-invasive procedure that can be carried out quickly. The collection of measurements for BMI is not specialised and does not require extensive training, nor is expensive equipment required. Additionally as BMI has been in use for such a long period of time, measurements collected in the present day can be compared to those going back over many generations.

### Other height to weight indices

As well as BMI there are other height and weight indices used as proxies for obesity. These include the Benn Index and the Ponderal Index. The Ponderal Index, also referred to as the Khosla-Lowe index, is similar to BMI but height is raised to the power of three, rather than two (mass/height$^3$). The Benn Index raises height to a population-specific exponent (mass/height$^P$), where P differs between samples. The means by which P is calculated from a sample is explained further in the original paper by Benn published in 1971.[49]

There is some suggestion that the Ponderal Index is suitable for neonates and should be used instead of birth weight, although some studies have suggested there is little difference between the two measures in predicting neonatal morbidity,[50,51] or that BMI is preferable.[52] The Ponderal Index is not thought to be a good measure for adiposity in adults.[53]

Amongst adults the Benn index and BMI have been suggested to be valid estimates of body fat in respect to their relationship with hydrostatic measures.[54] However, it is not evident that the population-specific exponent (P) in the Benn index conveys a material advantage in nutritional assessment,[55] and makes its use in public health and epidemiology complicated. It is not recommended for use in children.[56]

In general, BMI has supplanted all other weight and height indices as a measure of adiposity in all ages and has become the index of choice in measuring obesity.

### Abdominal circumference measurements

Waist circumference, measured at the midpoint between the lower border of the rib cage and the iliac crest, is found to be closely correlated to BMI, with both showing a similar association with future morbidity and mortality. Changes in waist circumference have been found to reflect changes in risk of comorbidities associated with obesity. This is particularly the case with cardiovascular disease (CVD) for which waist circumference is associated independently of BMI and may be a better predictor.[57–62] Waist circumference acts as a proxy measure of abdominal fat mass,[63,64] or total body fat.[65] Abdominal fat has been found to be of greater risk than fat deposited in other parts of the body, particularly when it is located within the abdominal cavity surrounding the organs, otherwise known as intra-abdominal or visceral fat. The WHO have outlined waist circumference measurements that denote enhanced relative risk (Table 1.2),[1] with different thresholds produced for men and women, as women show increases in relative risk of coronary heart disease (CHD) at lower waist circumferences than men.[66,67] These guidelines are also supported by the NHMRC, Australia[37] and in the United States for assessing abdominal adiposity.[39] However, abdominal fat mass can vary within a narrow range of total body fat or BMI due to other factors, with variation found between sexes,[68] by age[41,42] and ethnic group.[43]

Waist circumference when used on its own is uncontrolled for body shape, although there are a number of ratios used in order to allow this. Waist-to-hip or waist-to-height ratios provide some adjustment for the shape of the body, similar to BMI, and appear in some studies to be superior to waist circumference and BMI at predicting future disease risk.[69] NICE refer to a threshold for the waist-to-hip ratio of 1.0 for men and 0.85 for women, above which increased risk to health is indicated.[38]

The Conicity Index (CI) is an index that controls abdominal girth in metres by a function of weight in kilograms and height in metres[70] (Box 1.3). It has

---

**Box 1.3 Conicity Index**

$$CI = \frac{abdominal\ girth\ (metres)}{(0.109)\sqrt{\dfrac{Wt\ (kilograms)}{Ht\ (metres)}}}$$

---

**Table 1.2** Sex-specific waist circumference that denote increased risk of metabolic consequences

| SEX | RISK OF OBESITY-RELATED METABOLIC COMPLICATIONS | |
| --- | --- | --- |
| | Increased risk | Substantially increased risk |
| Men | ≥94 cm (≈37 inches) | ≥102 cm (≈40 inches) |
| Women | ≥80 cm (≈32 inches) | ≥88 cm (≈35 inches) |

been claimed that the CI has a number of advantages over waist-to- hip ratio as it has a theoretical range, it includes a built-in adjustment for height and weight and it does not require a measure of hip circumference.[70,71]

Although these indices provide some adjustment for the shape of the body, as well as appearing in some studies to be superior to waist circumference at predicting future disease risk,[62,72] it is unclear whether these measures alone can provide a superior indication of risk than BMI, despite proven links between measures of central adiposity and obesity-related ill health. NICE do not recommend using waist circumference as a routine measure, suggesting instead that circumference measures and ratios may be used to provide additional information on the risk of developing other long-term health problems.[38] WHO recommend thresholds to assess the relative risk of obesity-related ill health by combining BMI and waist circumference measurements (Table 1.3), in response to evidence that

an individual's relative risk of developing obesity-related health problems could be more accurately classified using both BMI and waist circumference than either measure alone.[1] These are recommended by both NICE[38] and NIH[39] in the USA with the NHMRC also recommending a combination of BMI and circumference measurements in assessing relative changes in fatness.[37] There are no evidence-based thresholds to classify individuals as being at increased risk using BMI with ratio measures such as waist-to-height or waist-to-hip.[62]

***Weaknesses and strengths of abdominal circumference measures***   A shared weakness of circumference measures is that both hip and waist measurements show greater degrees of intra- and inter-rater error than height and weight measurements and prove to be less accurate. Collecting circumference measures requires more extensive training to ensure the accuracy of the measurements. In comparison to BMI these measurements are also slightly more invasive, as measures

**Table 1.3** WHO classifications for risk of obesity-related ill health

| CLASSIFICATION | BMI (kg/m²) | WAIST CIRCUMFERENCE (cm) | |
|---|---|---|---|
| | | Normal WC* | Increased WC** |
| Underweight | <18.5 | No increased risk | No increased risk |
| Healthy weight | 18.5–24.9 | No increased risk | Increased risk |
| Overweight | 25–29.9 | Increased risk | High risk |
| Obesity | >30 | High risk | Very high risk |

*WC for Men 94–102; WC for women 80–88.
**WC for Men >102; WC for women >88.

of central adiposity generally require greater physical contact and involve the subject removing or lifting up outer clothing. This can make a difference in the obtaining of ethical consent for monitoring programmes and can make patients feel uneasy.

Despite concerns over the measurement process circumference measures are still relatively easy and cheap to obtain. They can be collected quickly and require little specialist training compared to most measures, excluding BMI. Evidence that circumference measures act as a proxy for abdominal fat and future ill health independently of BMI demonstrates that these measures provide additional information to BMI, hence recommendations to combine these measurements.

### Skinfold estimation methods

Skinfold estimation methods are based on skinfold thickness tests in which the thickness of subcutaneous fat located beneath the skin is measured by grasping a fold of skin and subcutaneous fat and measuring its thickness using calipers, at several standardised points on the body. These measurements are converted to an estimated body fat percentage by an equation. Some formulas require as few as three measurements, usually taken at the triceps, subscapular and supra-iliac sites,[38] others as many as seven.

**Weaknesses and strengths of skinfold estimation methods** It is very important when collecting skinfold

measures to test in a precise location with a fixed pressure, hence intra- and inter-rater reliability has been found to be an issue for skin fold measurement.[73] Although reliability can be improved by training and standardisation of technique this requires greater training than height, weight and circumference measures. Different results are possible with different methods, whilst the accuracy of these estimates is more dependent on a person's unique body fat distribution than on the number of sites measured. Skinfold measurements also involve body contact between operator and subject, normally requiring the removal of clothing, particularly from the upper part of the body, hence, measurement may be considered intrusive or embarrassing by some individuals. Skinfold-based body fat estimation is also sensitive to the type of caliper used; thus equipment must be standardised.

Skinfold estimation methods only measure subcutaneous adipose tissue, the fat located under the skin at particular points around the body. Individuals may have equal measurements at all skinfold sites, yet differ greatly in their body fat levels, in particular due to differences in fat deposits in other parts of the body such as visceral adipose tissue. Additionally, older individuals have been found to have a lower body density for the same skinfold measurements, assumed to signify a higher body fat percentage; however, older, highly athletic individuals might not fit this assumption, causing the formulas to underestimate their body density. Some models attempt to partially address many of these problems by including age as a variable in the statistics and the resulting formula.

Although skinfold measurements may not give an accurate reading of real body fat percentage, they can be used as a reliable measure of body composition change over a period of time, provided the test is carried out by the same person with the same technique to avoid intra- and inter-rater reliability concerns.[38]

### Bio Impedance Analysis

Bio Impedance Analysis (BIA) utilises the different electrical properties of lean tissue and adipose tissue in order to produce an estimate of an individual's percentage body fat. Lean tissue is made up of over 70% water and therefore acts as an electrical conductor, whereas adipose tissue has no water content acting as an insulator, therefore impeding the flow of electricity through the body. In order to produce an estimate for percentage body fat a low and safe electrical current is passed through the body using electrodes that are held or stood on by the individual and which also measure the impedance, or resistance to the flow of this current through the body. From these measures the BIA machine estimates total body water, then converting this into an estimate of body fat and fat-free mass (FFM) using prediction equations along with measurements of height, weight, age and sex, normally entered into the machine manually.[74] NICE do

not recommend using BIA as a substitute for BMI in measuring general adiposity,[38] whilst guidelines published in the United States also detail that BIA provides no advantage over BMI in the clinical management of patients, although these guidelines were published in 1998.[39] The NHMRC warn that BIA may be used in settings in which its limitations may not be understood by those operating it.[75]

**Weaknesses and strengths of Bio Impedance Analysis** Although small inexpensive BIA devices are available which measure impedance hand-to-hand or foot-to-foot, as well as being used whilst standing, there is concern that impedance measurements using these types of BIA devices are disproportionately determined by the tissues of the limbs that are in contact with the electrodes, meaning that they may fail to assess trunk adiposity accurately. Validations of old BIA devices suggest it is not as accurate as BMI in predicting body fat.[47]

Segmental BIA devices claim to include accurate measurements of abdominal adiposity by measuring the impedance of arms, legs and trunk separately. Segmental BIA is possible using devices individuals can stand on, providing electrodes for hands and feet. These devices are slightly more expensive and less portable than the more accessible machines and still may not completely account for abdominal fat. BIA devices have been developed that measure impedance of the abdominal region using an electrode belt, with the only additional input required being the sex of the participant. Tests on newer devices which attempt to measure the whole body indicate that these correlate well with total abdominal adipose tissue, although this correlation was not stronger than BMI measurements. It was also found that along with BMI and waist circumference, this particular BIA device which measures abdominal impedance did not provide a good proxy for visceral fat, suggesting that a more sophisticated imaging technique such as MRI is warranted when attempting to measure it.[48] Additionally this new device was found to be a precise measure of both abdominal fat and waist circumference, although it did not show any closer correlation with total body fat as determined by MRI than manual waist circumference measures and BMI.[76]

In general impedance readings can vary with skin conditions such as dryness, temperature and the presence of sweat such that individual differences in hydration state may confound the impedance readings. This can influence many measures, however, as hydration can also influence mass leading to changes in BMI. BIA is also not suitable for use on anyone with significant amounts of metal in the body (for example, joint replacements or pacemakers) or on pregnant women, who carry extra weight and extracellular water. Additionally few of the equations to estimate body fat from the impedance measurements have been developed in non-white populations[77]

so their validity when applied to populations other than those in which they were developed is unclear.

Although BIA devices take intricate measures of impedance, they are relatively easy to use and require little training, with some designed for home use. These devices can also be used to measure weight, or mass, and so can therefore be used at the same time to calculate BMI; therefore the additional collection of impedance data is of little imposition. It is also clear that much development has occurred within BIA in recent years. It is, therefore, possible that both the devices and equations used to calculate body fat percentage may improve, meaning that more accurate measures may be collected in the future and measurements which have already been collected could be converted to

---

**! Thinking points**

1. Classifying overweight and obesity uses very distinct cut-offs, how should these be used so that at-risk individuals are not missed?
2. If someone is not classified as obese through these measurements what else could be measured or discussed in order to identify any future risk?
3. What needs to be done to ensure that the measurements taken are reliable?
4. What makes a desirable measurement in investigating obesity on an individual and population level?

more accurate estimates of body fat through using these improved equations.

## Technical measures of obesity

A number of more technical and advanced means by which to measure obesity have been developed. These more technical means may prove to be more accurate that the more common methods described above but in general are more time consuming, more expensive and require specialist training. Technical measures are discussed below in terms of body density measures, chemical measures, internal scanning and photography and 3-D body scanning.

### Body density measurements

Body density measurements are normally obtained in two ways, either in water using a dunk tank, otherwise known as hydrodensitometry, or using air in a body pod, also known as air-displacement plethysmography.

Dunk tanks compare an individual's weight in water to their weight in air, whilst controlling for lung volume. Body tissues vary in their buoyancy with adipose tissue more buoyant than lean tissue. Individuals with proportionally higher body fat will therefore have less overall body density. Body pods measure the body volume of an individual by measuring the amount of air displaced by an individual. A body pod consists of two chambers, separated by a sensitive membrane that measures pressure. The change in air pressure in the test chamber between when it contains a person and when it does not are compared, and body volume is calculated. This measure of body volume can then be converted into a measure of body density by adjusting for the height and weight of the individual. These measures of body density can then be converted into percentage fat mass using a standard equation.[78]

### Weaknesses and strengths of body density measures

Both dunk tanks and body pods are expensive equipment that require specialist training. The dunk tank requires the participant to get wet, whilst for both methods, measurement requires individuals to wear a tight-fitting bathing suit, the body pod also requiring the wearing of a swim cap. Conditions such as temperature and humidity can affect the results and in the dunk tank individuals must be able to expire completely.[78] Although both provide a measure of body density, or body volume, rather than percentage fat mass, an equation is used to convert these measures into an estimate of percentage fat mass. However, this assumes consistent density in fat-free mass between individuals, which is not always the case, for example children's bones are less dense than adults, whereas athletes commonly have more dense bones than non-athletes.[78]

Both body density measurements have a high level of accuracy in collecting measurements, it is only in converting these into estimates for other measures such as percentage body fat that inaccuracies occur.

They can therefore be useful in comparing one measure, or monitoring one individual.

### Chemical measures

The two most common forms of chemical measures of obesity are isotope dilution and body cell counting. Isotope dilution uses a measure of body hydration to estimate total body fat. Healthy adults typically have a mean hydration of 73%. As adipose tissue has no water content, individuals with high adiposity will have a lower percentage hydration. To take the measurement a known quantity of isotope is ingested; one of three is commonly used: oxygen-18, deuterium, and tritium. After allowing for equilibration, a sample of body fluids, usually serum, is taken and the correlation of the isotope is then measured by mass spectroscopy or infrared methods providing a measurement of percentage of body fluids.[79] Body cell counting takes advantage of the known ratio of radioactive potassium $^{40}K$ to non-radioactive $^{39}K$. A measure of the radioactive isotope in an individual can be used to calculate total body potassium which can be used to derive an estimate of intracellular fluid and body cell mass,[80] if you assume a constant relationship between total body potassium and fat-free mass.[2] Total body fat is then calculated by subtracting the fat-free mass estimated from this measurement from the measured mass of the individual.

***Weaknesses and strengths of chemical measures*** Although some report isotope dilution as simple and inexpensive, others discuss the high cost and difficulty in mass spectrometer analysis;[81] potassium counting is also expensive in comparison to more simple methods and requires specialist training.[2] Isotope dilution assumes a constant relationship between total body weight and fat-free mass (0.73);[80] a general reference is also used in potassium counting which can vary by sex, ethnicity and age, particularly before and after puberty.[82] Additionally the radioactive measurement of potassium is carried out in a darkened room and can prove frightening for children.[81]

Both chemical measurements collect accurate chemical readings; if equations are accurate these can lead to precise measures of body fat. These can prove useful in monitoring individuals over time.

### Internal scanning

A number of methods can be used to take internal scans of the body to estimate body fat. These include dual-energy X-ray absorptiometry (DXA), computerised tomography (CT) and magnetic resonance imaging (MRI).

Dual-energy X-ray absorptiometry (DXA) uses X-ray absorption to estimate the amounts and densities of various tissues within the body, bone, muscle and fat, as they all transmit X-rays differently. Computerised tomography (CT) is a medical imaging method that produces a three-dimensional image of the inside of an individual by computerised digital geometry processing of a series of two-dimensional X-ray images taken around a single axis of rotation. Magnetic resonance imaging (MRI) uses powerful magnetic fields to produce three-dimensional images of the inside of an individual that provide a good contrast of the soft tissues of the body. Quantitative magnetic resonance (QMR), also known as ECHO MRI, is a relatively new technique that is recognised as an important recent development in the measurement of body composition.[61] QMR takes advantage of the varying nuclear magnetic resonance properties between the nuclei of hydrogen atoms in tissues with different chemical compositions. This allows QMR to differentiate signals from hydrogen atoms in fat, lean tissue and free water leading to measures of fat mass, lean mass and total body water.[83]

**Weaknesses and strengths of internal scans** All these forms of measurement require very expensive machinery that can only be used by extensively trained operators and interpreters. They are also very time consuming, in particular CT, MRI and QMR;[83] it can therefore be very difficult to undertake full body scans to allow a measure of total body fat. Additionally DXA only measures in two dimensions, so cannot be used to differentiate directly between visceral

and subcutaneous fat[84] and along with CT scans involve a relatively high radiation dose.[84,85] A validation of QMR suggests it may underestimate fat mass and overestimate lean mass, with these inaccuracies increasing with increasing body mass. The chambers in which participants sit in CT, MRI and QMR machines are fixed in size and although these can vary between machines it can be difficult to fit large patients into them and alternatives may need to be found.

CT scanning has been shown to be an accurate and precise technique for measuring soft tissue[86] and allows differentiation between visceral and subcutaneous fat in a cross-section of the body.[85] MRI compares well with CT for the measurement of body fat, allowing it to distinguish between subcutaneous and visceral fat; both techniques have a similar accuracy in comparison with chemical analysis. Internal scans such as MRI are recommended for quantifying visceral fat accurately which the more common methods of measurement are unable to do.[76] MRI scans use magnetic and radio waves, meaning that there is no exposure to ionising radiation such as with X-rays and CTs.

## Body imaging

Body imaging involves the use of digital image plethysmography (DIP) in which photographs from digital cameras are converted into a measure of body volume and/or produce a three-dimensional (3-D) body scan which attempts to record and measure body shape from which measurements of body volume along with lengths and circumferences can be extracted.[87,88] We discuss the three main types of 3-D body scanner: photogrammetric, laser and millimetre wave, all of which capture sophisticated raw data on body surface topography. DIP and 3-D body scanning traditionally involve booths, these can support cameras or light sensors surrounding a central space in which the subject must stand in a specified stance, unaided, for the duration of the scan; this can last approximately ten seconds in 3-D scanning to just under a minute for some DIP.[89] In general the equipment is expensive and large but it can be mobile, while the cost per scan is low. DIP equipment is usually cheaper than for the other 3-D scanners.

For DIP, one front and one lateral digital image of each subject are taken, the complete picture of the body is then used to produce an estimate of body volume known as dual digital photograph anthropometry.[89] Photogrammetric scanners project uniform patterns of visible light on to the body allowing cameras in the scanning booth to record the patterns, which have been distorted by the contours of the body.[88] The 3-D shape of the body is then inferred using spectroscopy. Laser scanners operate on similar principles as photogrammetric scanners in projecting safe, invisible lasers on to

the body whilst cameras that are offset from the laser source record the data. Triangulation methods are then used to calculate the location of the point or line.[87,88] Millimetre wave scanners are also known as ultrasonography or sonography, they use linear array radio waves to detect body shape.[87,88]

**Weaknesses and strengths of imaging**  3-D scanners and DIP acquisition share the principles of capturing and analysing information about body shape and therefore share the same criticisms that it is uncertain whether body shape can be used to classify obesity-related ill-health without taking into account fat distribution or body composition. Equipment is expensive for all forms of scanning, but although the equipment for DIP acquisition is less expensive than that used in 3-D body scanning the subjects must stand still, unaided, for a longer period of time. DIP, photogrammetric and laser scanning require the subject to strip down to tight-fitting underwear or a bathing suit and for weight measurements to be taken. Laser scanning is also most accurate if participants hold their breath after maximum expiration.[90] Validation of laser scanning against other methods of volume measurement have not supported their use in predicting adiposity for adults[91] with no validation attempted with children. It is also thought that the data collected by millimetre wave scanners may be less accurate compared with photogrammetric or laser scanners because water under the skin causes distortion.[87,88]

For some forms of scanning as this process is almost entirely automated, little operator skill is required after some initial training. The final 3-D scanned images may also be used to obtain circumference measures for a variety of places on the body, permitting the calculation of waist measurements and ratios. One advantage of the millimetre wave scanners over the other types discussed here is that they can scan through clothing.

---

### ⚠ Thinking points

1. What advantages do these technical measures of obesity have over more common methods?
2. When should we use these more technical measures of obesity?
3. What attributes should future technological measurements include if they are to be used on a large-scale basis?
4. MRI scans provide an accurate internal scan of an individual, clearly demonstrating fat distribution. Why can we not use this for every patient?

---

### Classifying obesity in children

Much less validation has been performed on the methods to classify weight status in children than in adults. Many of the technical methods described above are not suitable for use with children, in particular those that require the participant to remain stationary for an extended period of time, or those with specialist equipment that may seem intimidating for younger participants. Of the more common methods used to measure obesity, differences between individuals in growth rates by age, sex and ethnic group mean that the use of skinfold thickness[44] and BIA[92] should be interpreted with caution, and it is imperative that specialist equations are used for converting measurements to estimates for body fat.

There are also no evidence-based thresholds for waist circumference measurements in children. The relationship between waist circumference and adiposity for children will change with age; therefore, it is not possible to use a fixed set of thresholds as is done with adults. Suggestions have been made that a waist-to-height ratio of 0.5 or greater may prove a useful threshold for increased disease risk for children; however, more research is needed in this area before this is accepted.[72]

As with adults, BMI is the most commonly used measure for classifying weight status in children; however, its use in children is more complicated due to the changes in growth that occur during the childhood years. To account for this, thresholds that vary by age and sex are created such that weight status can be classified at different levels over the course of childhood and between the sexes. These thresholds are commonly referred to as child growth reference curves.

There are a number of different child growth references available and used internationally, derived from different reference populations. By collecting height and weight from reference populations, curves depicting how BMI varies by age and sex are created. From this the distribution of the average BMI by age for both sexes is created, and weight status defined by deviance from this mean either by standard deviation or by centile of the reference population.

The choice of which growth curves to use is normally influenced by protocol within that country, for example NICE recommend specific thresholds from the UK90 growth curves; the CDC and NHMRC recommend the use of the CDC charts; whereas the International Obesity Task Force (IOTF) has developed charts for international use. It is crucial when using a growth reference curve to classify obesity in a sample or population, that comparisons to this are only made using the same thresholds, as different thresholds will result in different classifications and therefore prevalence. The most commonly used growth references are:

### 1. British 1990 growth reference (UK90)

NICE recommend using the British 1990 growth reference (UK90) for population monitoring and clinical assessment in children aged four years and over[38] in the UK, although other BMI thresholds can be used in particular for international comparison of obesity prevalence.

The UK90 BMI reference provides centile curves for BMI for British children from birth to 23 years. They are based on a sample of 32,222 measurements from 12 distinct surveys collected between 1978 and 1994.[93,94] The BMI reference curves are part of the wider British 1990 growth reference which also includes height, weight, head circumference and waist circumference;[95] however, there are currently no recommended centile thresholds to grade children as being at increased risk from waist circumference and attempts to generate them are thought to require validation.[96]

The UK90 BMI reference is available on printed growth charts, and depicts centiles evenly spaced at 2/3 of a standard deviation. The centiles displayed on the UK90 growth charts are: 0.4th, 2nd, 9th, 25th, 50th, 75th, 91st, 98th and 99.6th. Different thresholds are recommended for population monitoring and clinical assessment; 85th and 95th centiles determine overweight and obese status respectively for population monitoring whilst 91st and 98th are used for clinical assessment (Table 1.4). This means only those for clinical assessment are depicted in the chart. NICE recommend tailored clinical intervention for children with a BMI at or above the 91st centile and assessment of comorbidity for those at or above the 98th centile.[38]

### 2. International Obesity Task Force (IOTF) cut-offs

The IOTF thresholds have been promoted for use internationally and are therefore most commonly used when making international

**Table 1.4** NICE thresholds for weight status in children using the UK90 growth charts

|  | POPULATION MONITORING | CLINICAL ASSESSMENT |
| --- | --- | --- |
| Underweight | 2nd centile | 2nd centile |
| Overweight | 85th centile | 91st centile |
| Obese | 95th centile | 98th centile |

comparisons, or when presenting findings to an international audience.

They have been derived from body mass index data from six large, nationally representative, cross-sectional surveys from Brazil, Great Britain, Hong Kong, the Netherlands, Singapore and the United States, and they cover ages from 2 to 18 years. Each of these surveys consisted of more than 10,000 subjects and covered ages of at least 6 to 18 years. The total sample when combining these surveys included 192,727 individuals aged 0 to 25 years.

The International Obesity Task Force (IOTF) thresholds have been derived to line up with the adult BMI thresholds for obesity and overweight at age 18 years, with underweight defined from equivalent adult BMIs of 16, 17 and 18.5.[95]

### 3. World Health Organization (WHO) Child Growth Standard

The WHO Child Growth Standard is recommended for use internationally with children aged 0 to 5 years. These growth standards are also recommended for use in the UK with children 4 years and under.

The WHO Child Growth Standard is based on an international sample

from Brazil, Ghana, India, Norway, Oman and the United States, totalling 26,985 measurements of weight and length for those aged 0 to 24 months, and weight and height for those aged 24 to 71 months.

WHO suggest a set of thresholds by sex based on single standard deviation spacing. These thresholds include length or height for age; weight for age; weight for length; weight for height and BMI for age.[95]

### 4. World Health Organization (WHO) 2007 growth reference

The WHO 2007 growth reference is recommended internationally for children aged 5 to 19 years. These curves were derived from a combination of the USA National Center for Health Statistics 1977 pooled growth data, and the WHO Multi-centre Growth Reference Study (MGRS) from Brazil, Ghana, Norway, India, Oman and USA.

The WHO 2007 reference aligns with the WHO Child Growth Standards at age five years and is available for height, weight and BMI for age.[95]

Thresholds for weight status are set on standard deviation spacing from the average:

- Underweight = <−2 standard deviations (SD).
- Overweight = +1 SD to +2 SD.
- Obese>2 SD.

### United States Centers for Disease Control and Prevention (CDC) 2000 growth reference

The CDC 2000 growth reference is primarily used in the United States with children and young people aged 2 to 20 years; it is also recommended for use in Australia by the NHMRC.[75] It was derived from a sample population from the United States consisting of a number of national health examination surveys with supplementary information collected from birth certificates and hospital data on child birth weight, length, and head circumference.

The CDC 2000 growth reference defines children at risk of overweight and obesity if their BMI exceeds the 85th and 95th centiles for most routine assessments. The 90th and 97th centiles are used for special health care requirements. The third and fifth centiles are used to define underweight status.[95] See Box 1.4 for online information on growth charts.

### Adiposity rebound

The development of adipose tissue within an individual commonly comprises of a number of phases, one of which is known as the adiposity rebound.

---

**Box 1.4 Online information on growth charts**

UK90 – www.healthforallchildren.co.uk

UK WHO growth charts for 0 to 4 years of age – http://www.rcpch.ac.uk/growthcharts

IOTF charts – www.bmj.com/content/320/7244/1240.abstract

WHO Growth Standard – www.who.int/childgrowth/standards/

WHO 2007 growth reference – www.who.int/growthref/en/

CDC 2000 growth reference – www.cdc.gov/growthcharts/cdc_charts.htm

---

During the first year of life adiposity increases rapidly due to the growth in the size of the adipose cells, otherwise known as adipocytes, which then diminish over the next year or two.[97–99] Over this period of decreasing adiposity, although the adipose cell number remains stable, body height continues to increase which leads to an apparent slimming of the child. After a number of years during which there is stability in the number of adipose cells, there is a second period of rapid growth in body fat, commonly starting at around 6 years of age. The minimum value of BMI throughout a child's development, due to the increase in height and stability in adiposity, occurs just before this second period of growth, known as the adiposity rebound, a phrase first coined in 1984.[99]

From this moment, both the size and number of adipocytes increase,[97–99]

leading to an increase in BMI due to an accelerated deposition of weight which is driven by more rapid accumulation of body fat rather than lean tissue mass[100,101] and no slowing of height gain.[100,102] Growth reference curves demonstrate this event through an increase after the lowest point on the curve,[99,103–106] suggesting an age at which the average child will undergo adiposity rebound with children undergoing an early rebound thought to be at a greater risk of future obesity and obesity-related ill health.[99]

The timing of adiposity rebound in children has therefore been suggested by some as a means by which to identify children at risk from obesity-related ill health. It has been proposed that an early age at adiposity rebound predicts later fatness, as it identifies children whose body mass index centile is high and/or crossing upward, with children with an early rebound having a greater risk of later obesity.[100,107–113] Further evidence suggests that it is associated with a higher risk of obesity-related future ill health including diabetes[100,114,115] and elevated blood pressure, although it should be recognised that this is not a universal finding.[100]

Identifying early rebound in young children may, therefore, be used to identify children at risk, enabling strategies to be put in place that can limit excessive fat gain and the later development of obesity.[107] Adiposity rebound has not been accepted by all as a clinical tool.[100] The mechanisms underlying the increased risks associated with an early adiposity rebound have yet to be determined[100,116] and the time frame required for a measurement of rebound that is predictive is not higher than that of a single BMI measurement in mid-childhood.[100,102] However, waiting until a child is 7 or 8 years of age if they have demonstrated a very early rebound could miss a valuable opportunity to intervene.[100] Certainly regardless of the clinical applicability of adiposity rebound, improving our understanding of what controls the dynamics of childhood body composition and mechanisms that delay adiposity rebound could help prevent obesity by expanding our ability to manage the increasing problem of fat gain during childhood growth.[100,117]

---

## ! Thinking points

1. Why are growth charts used with children instead of general cut-offs as with adults?
2. How will you decide which growth chart to use for classifying obesity in children?
3. Why is it challenging to use the same growth curves with children from different ethnic backgrounds?
4. What other factors should you consider when assessing obesity risk in children?

**Summary points**

- Obesity is a medical condition characterised by excess body fat.
- The WHO recommends the measuring of individuals to assess individual risk of obesity.
- Screening programmes are accompanied by an explicit intention to treat overweight and obese individuals.
- Surveillance programmes are used to measure prevalence and monitor trends over time.
- BMI is a quick and easy tool for classifying obesity risk in large numbers of individuals and a high BMI has a proven link to ill health.
- BMI does not distinguish between lean and adipose tissue, nor does it provide an estimation of abdominal adipose tissue.
- It is recommended that circumference measurements are used alongside BMI but not instead of.
- Technical measures may provide more accurate measurement of body fat, but are more expensive, require specialist training and take more time than more common measures.
- Internal scans, in particular MRI, provide measures of fat distribution that can identify levels of visceral fat.
- Using BMI to classify weight status for children requires the use of growth curves which make adjustments for sex and age.
- There are a number of recommended growth charts, with their use determined by either the protocol within countries or the aims of any analysis.
- The absence of age- and sex-specific thresholds for circumference measures amongst children makes it difficult to use these measures for these age groups.
- Early adiposity rebound may be used to identify children at risk from future obesity-related ill health.

## Web pages and resources

Australian Government National Health and
    Medical Research Council (NHMRC).
www.nhmrc.gov.au/research/obesity.
Centers for Disease Control and Prevention (CDC).
www.cdc.gov/obesity/.
NHS choices.
www.nhs.uk/Conditions/Obesity/Pages/
    Introduction.aspx.
The WHO regional office for Europe.
www.euro.who.int/en/what-we-do/health-topics/
    noncommunicable-diseases/obesity.
The Public Health England Obesity Knowledge
    and Intelligence team.
www.noo.org.uk/.

## Further reading

1. WHO. Obesity and Overweight. Factsheet
   No. 311, Geneva: World Health Organization;
   Last updated 2011. http://www.who.int/
   mediacentre/factsheets/fs311/en/.
   *This factsheet produced by the WHO introduces the
   concepts and definitions of overweight and obesity.
   It goes on to describe recommended measurements,
   also discussing some of the consequences and causes
   of obesity.*
2. Browning, et al. Measuring abdominal adipose
   tissue: comparison of simpler methods
   with MRI. Obes Facts 2011;4:9–15. http://
   content.karger.com/produktedb/produkte.
   asp?DOI=000324546&typ=pdf.

This is a cross-sectional study that compares the measurement of visceral and total abdominal adipose tissue by magnetic resonance imaging (MRI) against a range of 'simpler' techniques: BMI, waist circumference (WC), bioelectrical impedance (BIA) devices and dual X-ray absorptiometry (DXA).

3. NOO. A Simple Guide to Classifying Body Mass Index in Children. Oxford: National Obesity Observatory; 2011.

http://www.noo.org.uk/uploads/doc/vid_11762_classifyingBMIinchildren.pdf. This briefing paper produced by NOO provides a simple guide to how body mass index (BMI) can be used to assess the weight status of children. It describes the different growth curves that can be used to interpret BMI in children and young people, explains how they differ, and where they are commonly used.

# Obesity prevalence and trends

There are a number of surveillance programmes which describe prevalence figures for obesity measurements on a national level. Data from these surveys are drawn on to present the most recent figures at the time of publication in the UK and Ireland, North America and Australasia.

## UK and Ireland prevalence figures

### England

***Adult prevalence*** The 2010 *Health Survey for England (HSE)* found that for adults aged 16 years and over, 26.2% of men and 26.1% of women were obese; additionally 67.8% of men and 57.8% of women were overweight or obese. It also reports that 34.2% of men and 46.4% of women have a raised waist circumference, whilst only 42.0% of men and 41.1% of women have no increased risk using the BMI and waist circumference WHO classifications; see Table 2.1.[1]

***Child prevalence*** The 2010 HSE also describes prevalence amongst children using the UK90 thresholds. Amongst boys aged 2 to 15 years, 17.1% were classified as obese and 31.4% were overweight or obese. For girls of the same age, the figures were 14.8% and 29.2% respectively.[1]

*The National Child Measurement Programme (NCMP)* collects data from large numbers of children in two primary school year groups in England every year. Prevalence figures from the most recent programme can be found in Table 2.2. These come from the 2010/11 academic year and use UK90 growth charts to determine BMI status.[2]

Both the HSE and the NCMP collect measured height and weight from which BMI is calculated. The HSE also collects waist circumference measurements for adults. This allows raised waist circumference and the WHO classification of increased risk to be calculated.

*The Health Survey for England (HSE)* is a series of annual surveys designed

**Table 2.1** Prevalence of WHO classifications for adults in England, Health Survey for England 2010

| RISK CATEGORY | MEN (%) | WOMEN (%) |
|---|---|---|
| Not applicable | 1.1 | 1.5 |
| No increased risk | 42.0 | 41.1 |
| Increased risk | 21.7 | 13.8 |
| High risk | 12.3 | 18.9 |
| Very high risk | 22.8 | 24.6 |

*Source: Health Survey for England 2010 Copyright © 2012, Re-used with the permission of The Health and Social Care Information Centre. All rights reserved.*

**Table 2.2** Prevalence of BMI status for children in England, NCMP 2010/11

| YEAR GROUP | SEX | OBESE (%) | OVERWEIGHT AND OBESE (%) |
|---|---|---|---|
| Reception (4 to 5 years of age) | Boys | 10.1 | 23.9 |
| | Girls | 8.8 | 21.4 |
| Year 6 (10 to 11 years of age) | Boys | 20.6 | 34.9 |
| | Girls | 17.4 | 31.8 |

*Source: National Health Service Information Service 2012. National Childhood Measurement Programme, England, school year 2010/11.*

to measure health and health-related behaviours in adults and children in England. It has a series of core elements that are included every year and special topics that are included in selected years. Anthropometric measurements are included in the core topics, and so BMI and obesity data are produced for every year of the survey. Details on the HSE, along with publications and data can be found at the National Health Service (NHS) Information Centre (IC) website: www.ic.nhs.uk

Details on the *National Child Measurement Programme (NCMP)* can be found in the Case Study in Chapter 1 (Box 1.1). Information and publications on the NCMP can be found through the NHS Information Centre website: www.ic.nhs.uk. Further information and publications can be found through the Public Health England Obesity Knowledge and Intelligence team website who publish users' guides for those people wishing to use NCMP data as well as providing interactive e-atlases, in which NCMP data for all years of the study can be presented for different regions in England and mapped against other regional measures: www.noo.org.uk.

## Scotland

**Adult prevalence** The 2010 *Scottish Health Survey (SHeS)* reports that for adults over the age of 16 years, 27.4% of men and 28.9% of women are obese whilst 67.8% of men and 62.4% of women are overweight or obese.[3]

**Child prevalence** For children aged 2 to 15 years, according to UK90 growth charts, 15.6% of boys were obese and 31.1% overweight or obese; for girls of the same age the figures were 12.9% and 28.5% respectively.[3]

The SHeS collects measured height and weight data that are converted into BMI. The Scottish Health Survey was introduced in 1995 with data collections in 1995, 1998 and 2003. The continuous Scottish Health Survey began in January 2008 and ran continuously from 2008 to 2011. An annual report is published for each year of the survey, whilst a contract has recently been awarded to continue the survey for a further four years from 2012 to 2015. Information on the SHeS along with publications and statistics can be found through the Scottish Executive Government website: www.scotland.gov.uk

## Wales

**Adult prevalence** Results from the 2010 *Welsh Health Survey (WHS)* estimate that for adults aged 16 years and above 22% of men and 21% of women were obese and 63% of men and 52% of women were overweight or obese.[4]

**Child prevalence** Using UK90 growth charts for children aged 2 to 15 years the WHS found that 23% of boys were obese and 38% overweight or obese, whilst 16% of girls were obese and 34% overweight or obese.[4]

The WHS collects self-reported height and weight data rather than measured data. The WHS was established in October 2003 and is an annual survey that runs all year round. The WHS is commissioned by the Welsh Assembly Government to provide information about the health of people in Wales. NatCena, a not-for-profit independent social research organisation, has been involved in the survey since its inception. Information, publications and data from the WHS can be found through the Welsh Assembly Government website: wales.gov.uk

## Northern Ireland

**Adult prevalence** The 2005/06 Northern Ireland *Health and Social Wellbeing Survey* found that for adults 16 years and older 25% of men and 23% of women were obese, whilst 64% of men and 53% of women were overweight or obese.[5] In 2010/11 the Health Survey Northern Ireland reported that 23% of men and women were obese, with 77% of men overweight and obese compared to 53% of women.[6]

**Child prevalence** Using UK90 growth charts data from the 2005/06 *Northern Ireland Health and Wellbeing*

*Survey* found that for children aged 2 to 15 years, 20% of boys were obese and 39% overweight or obese, whilst 15% of girls were obese and 31% were overweight or obese.[5] The 2010/11 Health Survey Northern Ireland presented child prevalence figures determined by the International Obesity Task Force (IOTF) growth curves, suggesting that 8% of boys and 9% of girls were obese, whilst a similar percentage of both sexes were overweight or obese (27%).[6]

The *Northern Ireland Health and Social Wellbeing Survey (NIHSWS)* was commissioned by the Department of Health, Social Services and Public Safety and commissioned the Northern Ireland Statistics and Research Agency (NISRA) to conduct the fieldwork for the survey. The survey was conducted in 1997, 2001 and 2005/06. Information, results and publications can be found through the NISRA website: www.csu.nisra.gov.uk

The *Health Survey Northern Ireland* is a new Department of Health, Social Services and Public Safety survey that will run every year on a continuous basis; 2010/11 was the first year of data collection.

Information on this survey can be found through the Department of Health, Social Services and Public Safety website: www.dhsspsni.gov.uk

## Ireland

***Adult prevalence*** Measured data from the 2007 *Survey of Lifestyle, Attitudes and Nutrition in Ireland (SLÁN)* found that for adults aged 18 years and above, 24% of men and 26% of women were obese, whilst 69% of men and 59% of women were overweight and obese. The SLÁN also collected self-reported height and weight statistics, which reported that 16% of men and 13% of women were obese, with 59% of men and 41% of women overweight or obese, lower than for measured prevalence.[7] The 2011 *National Adult Nutrition Survey* found that for adults aged 18 years and above 45.7% of men and 33.3% of women were obese, whilst 71.3% of men and 55% of women were overweight or obese.[8]

***Child prevalence*** The 2005 National Children's Food Survey using UK90 growth charts found that for children aged 5 to 12 years, 11.1% were obese and 22.2% overweight and obese.[8] The 2008 National Teen's Food Survey also using UK90 growth charts found that for boys aged 13 to 17 years, 8.5% were obese and 19.3% were overweight or obese; for girls of the same age, 6.5% were obese and 17.6% overweight or obese.[8]

In the 2007 SLÁN self-reported BMIs were calculated for 9735 respondents whilst only 2174 respondents had their height and weight measured by a trained interviewer. The National Adult Nutrition Survey collected measurements of height, weight, waist circumference and hip circumference from which a range of anthropometric measurements could be published.

The 2007 Survey of Lifestyle, Attitudes and Nutrition in Ireland (SLÁN) was funded by the Health Promotion Policy Unit of the Department of Health and Children. The survey and analyses were carried out by the SLÁN 2007 Consortium, consisting of the Royal College of Surgeons in Ireland (RCSI), the National University of Ireland, Cork (UCC), the National University of Ireland, Galway (NUIG) and the Economic and Social Research Institute (ESRI). SLÁN surveys have been carried out in 1998, 2002 and 2007. Information and publications on SLÁN can be found through the Irish Social Science Data Archive (ISSDA) website: www.ucd.ie/issda/

The 2011 *National Adult Nutrition Survey*, the 2008 *National Teen's Food Survey* and the 2005 *National Children's Food Survey* are part of the National Nutrition Surveys programme carried out by the Irish Universities Nutrition Alliance (IUNA). IUNA is made up of four academic nutrition units from University College Cork, University of Ulster, Trinity College Dublin and University College Dublin. Information, publications and data from the National Nutrition Surveys can be found through the IUNA website: www.iuna.net

### Access to UK data on obesity

The British Heart Foundation (BHF) Heart statistics programme collects the most comprehensive and up-to-date statistics on the effects, prevention, treatment and causes of heart disease in the UK, including obesity and obesity-related risk factors such as dietary choice and physical activity. These statistics are available through publications, web-tables and figures all of which can be accessed through the Heart statistics website found via the BHF website: http://www.bhf.org.uk/research/statistics.aspx

Many of the datasets of the UK-based surveys can be accessed for use, including secondary analysis, through the Economic and Social Data Service (ESDS) including the HSE, SHeS, WHS, NIHSWS and aggregated data from the NCMP. The ESDS is a national data archiving and dissemination service which came into operation in January 2003. The service is a jointly funded initiative sponsored by the Economic and Social Research Council (ESRC) and the Joint Information Systems Committee (JISC). More information and access can be found through the ESDS website: www.esds.ac.uk/

## North America

### United States of America

*Adult prevalence*  In the USA the National Health and Nutrition Examination Survey (NHANES) data from 2009–2010 suggest that for adults older than 20 years of age 35.5% of men and 35.8% of women are obese.[9] Data from the 2007–2010 NHANES reports that 73.3% of men and 63.9% of women are overweight or obese.[10]

**Child prevalence** Data from the 2009–2010 NHANES reports prevalence for children as defined by the CDC 2000 growth charts, finding that for children aged two to 19 years 18.6% of boys were obese, whilst 33.0% were overweight or obese; for girls 15.0% were obese and 30.4% overweight or obese.[9]

The NHANES collects measured data on height and weight as well as other anthropometric data including circumference of the waist and mid-arm and skinfold thickness measurements.

The *National Health and Nutrition Examination Survey (NHANES)* is a programme of studies designed to assess the health and nutritional status of adults and children in the United States. NHANES is a major programme of the National Center for Health Statistics (NCHS), part of the Centers for Disease Control and Prevention (CDC) and has the responsibility for producing vital and health statistics for the nation. The NHANES programme began in the early 1960s and has been conducted as a series of surveys focusing on different population groups or health topics. In 1999, the survey became a continuous programme that has a changing focus on a variety of health and nutrition measurements to meet emerging needs. The survey examines a nationally representative sample of about 5000 persons each year. These persons are located in counties across the country, 15 of which are visited each year. The CDC provides more information and results from the NHANES online: www.cdc.gov/nchs/nhanes.htm

## Canada

**Adult prevalence** The 2007–2009 Canadian Health Measures Survey (CHMS) found that for men aged 18 to 79 years 23.9% were obese and 68.0% were overweight or obese; for women these figures were 23.6% and 53.1% respectively.[11]

**Child prevalence** The same survey found that according to IOTF thresholds for children aged 6 to 17 years, 10.0% of boys and 7.1% of girls were obese, whilst 27.0% of boys were overweight or obese compared to 24.4% of girls.[11]

The CHMS collects anthropometry measurements including standing height, sitting height, weight, waist circumference, hip circumference and skinfolds thickness. The *Canadian Health Measures Survey (CHMS)* was launched in 2007 and is being conducted by Statistics Canada in partnership with Health Canada and the Public Health Agency of Canada. Information, publications and data from the CHMS can be found at the Statistics Canada website: www.statcan.gc.ca

## Australasia

### Australia

**Adult prevalence** The 2007/08 Australian Bureau of Statistics (ABS) National Health Survey (NHS) reported measured data that found that for adults over 18 years of age 25.5% of men and 23.6% of women were obese and 67.2% of men and 54.6% of women were overweight or obese. The survey also collected self-reported data for adults that found 22.3% of men and 20.3% of women were obese whilst 63.6% of men and 48.3% of women were overweight or obese. All self-reported prevalence figures were lower than those from measured data.[12]

**Child prevalence** The 2007/08 NHS also reported that for children 5 to 17 years of age, 9.3% of boys and 5.6% of girls were obese, whilst 25.5% and 19.5% were overweight or obese respectively.

The 1995 and 2007/08 NHS collected measured height and weight information; other years of the survey only collected self-reported data.[12]

The *National Health Survey (NHS)* is conducted by the Australian Bureau of Statistics (ABS) with the 2007/08 survey the fifth in the series. Previous surveys in the series were conducted in 1989–90, 1995, 2001 and 2004–2005. Commencing with the 2001 survey, the survey is now conducted every three years. Health surveys conducted by the ABS in 1977–78 and 1983, while not part of the NHS series, also collected similar information. Information, publications and data from the NHS can be obtained through the Australian Bureau of Statistics' website: www.abs.gov.au

The Australian Bureau of Statistics (ABS), in close consultation with the

Department of Health and Ageing, is currently conducting the *Australian Health Survey*. This started in April 2011 and will run till 2013. No data from this were available at the time of publication. More information on this can be obtained through the Australian Bureau of Statistics website: www.abs.gov.au

## New Zealand

**Adult prevalence** The 2011/12 *New Zealand Health Survey (NZHS)* found that for adults over 15 years of age 28.1% of men and 28.8% of women were obese and 68.3% of men and 59.5% of women were overweight or obese.[13] The 2008/09 New Zealand Adult Nutrition Survey (NZANS) found among New Zealanders aged 15 years and over that 27.7% of men and 27.8% of women were obese whilst 69.0% of men and 60.6% of women were overweight or obese.[14]

**Child prevalence** Using IOTF cut offs, the 2011/12 NZHS found that for children aged 2 to 14 years 10.2% of boys and 10.2% of girls were obese, whilst 29.4% of boys were overweight or obese compared to 30.9% of girls.[62]

Both the NZHS and the NZANS collect measured height, weight and waist circumference.

The Health and Disability Intelligence (HDI) group within the Ministry of Health's Policy Business Unit is responsible for the design, analyses and reporting of the NZHS which has been run as part of a wider health survey programme that included a number of surveys. From 2011 these surveys have been integrated into the single NZHS, which is in continuous operation. The NZHS dress rehearsal went into the field in May 2011, and the NZHS then went into full operation in July 2011, with initial findings published in December 2012. Information, publications and data from the NZHS can be found through the New Zealand Ministry of Health website: www.health.govt.nz

The *New Zealand Adult Nutrition Survey (NZANS)* is a component of the New Zealand Health Monitor, an integrated programme of household surveys and cohort studies managed by the Ministry of Health and is a key element of the cross-sector programme of Official Social Statistics. The 2008/09 NZANS is the fourth national population-based nutrition survey in adults and the second funded by the Ministry of Health. Information, publications and data from the NZANS can be found through the New Zealand Ministry of Health website: www. health.govt.nz

---

**Thinking points**

1. Why can prevalence figures from national surveys not be used as exact figures of national prevalence?
2. Some surveys collect both self-reported and measured data, with measured data collected from fewer individuals; which of these provides a better estimate of national prevalence?
3. In some countries more than one programme collects prevalence data on obesity; what factors should be considered in choosing which programme provides the best estimate?
4. Some programmes collect a range of anthropometric measurements; what will influence which of these should be used?

---

# International prevalence of obesity

Comparing between countries in prevalence figures can be difficult. This requires utilising many sources of data. A number of organisations currently compile data on obesity from different countries and make these readily available to allow international comparisons to be made. These include the World Health Organization (WHO), the Organisation for Economic Co-operation and Development (OECD) and the International Association for the Study of Obesity (IASO). Details on these are provided below.

## WHO Global Health Observatory (apps.who.int/ghodata)

**Details** The GHO data repository provides access to over 50 datasets on priority health topics including overweight and obesity. It also provides on-line access to WHO's annual summary of health-related data for its 194 Member states. For many countries estimates have been calculated to compare between countries and across time. Where data are not available for a country, estimates are modelled using data from other countries and specific country characteristics.

*Data available:*
  Prevalence overweight
  (BMI ≥ 25 kg/m²)
  Prevalence obese (BMI ≥ 30 kg/m²)
  Mean body mass index trends
  1980–2008 (crude estimate)
  Mean body mass index trends
  1980–2008 (age standardised
  estimate)
*Demographics:*
  By sex
  Adults ≥ 20 years of age

## WHO Global Infobase (https://apps.who.int/infobase/Comparisons.aspx)

**Details**  The WHO Global InfoBase is a data warehouse that collects, stores and displays information on chronic diseases and their risk factors for all WHO member states as well as presenting maps and graphs of these data. Data can be compared between countries or profiles on individual countries can be produced. So that the data are comparable, adjustments are made for differences between surveys for a number of factors including age distribution and year of data collection.

*Data available:*
  Prevalence overweight
  (BMI ≥ 25 kg/m²)
  Prevalence obese (BMI ≥ 30 kg/m²)
  Mean body mass index
*Demographics:*
  By sex
  Adults ≥ 15–100 years or
  30–100 years for all countries
  Age breakdown further for some
  countries

## WHO Global database on body mass index (http://apps.who.int/bmi)

**Details**  The WHO Global database provides both national and subnational adult underweight, overweight and obesity prevalence rates by country, year of survey and sex. The information is presented interactively as maps, tables, graphs and downloadable documents. The national level BMI data have been verified so that they apply to internationally recommended BMI cut-off points; however, the data presented are not directly comparable since they vary in terms of sampling procedures, age ranges and year of data collection. Subnational data are also available for some countries.

*Data available:*
Prevalence of a number of BMI categories including:
  Underweight (BMI ≤ 18.5 kg/m²)
  Normal weight (BMI 18.5–24.99 kg/m²)
  Overweight (BMI ≥ 25 kg/m²)
  Obese (BMI ≥ 30 kg/m²)
  Years 1960–2009

*Demographics:*
By sex
Adults aged ≥ 16 years for all
countries
Further age breakdown varies by
country

## OECD StatExtracts – Health Stats (www.oecd.org)

**Details** The Organisation for Economic Co-operation and Development (OECD), which provides statistics on overweight and obesity from 32 of the 34 member countries, displays a range of data from different years and that is both self-reported and measured.

*Data available:*
Prevalence of overweight
(BMI ≥ 25 kg/m$^2$)
Prevalence of obese (BMI ≥ 30 kg/m$^2$)
Data separated into self-report and measured
Years 1978–2010 but varies between countries
*Demographics:*
By sex
Adults aged ≥ 16 years for all countries

## IASO Obesity Data (www.iaso.org)

**Details** The International Association for the Study of Obesity (IASO) provides a range of data related to obesity. This includes data for children and adolescents as well as adults. Data are presented globally and for European Union countries. Not all data presented are age standardised, and due to varying methodologies are not always directly comparable. Prevalence figures are based on the best available data for the country; in some circumstances the data may be based on subnational surveys. Sources and references are available from IASO. Maps and charts describing prevalence figures are also available.

*Data available:*
Prevalence of overweight
(BMI ≥ 25 kg/m$^2$)
Prevalence of obese (BMI ≥ 30 kg/m$^2$)
Trends are available for both children and adults.
*Demographics:*
By sex
Data available for children, adolescents and adults

# Adult international prevalence

Comparing between countries in obesity prevalence can be problematic due to differences in the year of the most recent data, the populations studied and the measurement methodologies. The Organisation for Economic Co-operation and Development (OECD) which provides statistics on overweight and obesity from 32 of the 34 member countries displays a range of data from different years and stratifies this into self-reported and measured. Inspection of these data indicates that those countries collecting measured data have a higher prevalence of obesity than those collecting self-reported data, although it is impossible to ignore that self-reported measures have been found to lead to under-reported BMI.[15]

Some organisations including the WHO Global Infobase and the WHO Global Health Observatory attempt to control for these differences by standardising and adjusting data by factors such as sex distribution, age distribution and year of data collection to make them more comparable. In fact the WHO Global Health Observatory goes one step further by calculating estimates for countries which provide no data by using data from other countries and any specific country characteristics that are available. This means that data presented by these organisations are different from the survey data collected within the country and vary from other organisations that use the same data but make little or no adjustments, such as the IASO. In Tables 2.3 and 2.4, a selection of countries which are found to have the highest adult prevalence figures in men and women are presented for both IASO and WHO Global Infobase

**Table 2.3** Top five countries and selected other countries for obesity prevalence (BMI >30 kg/m²) in males and selected other countries, IASO 2012 and WHO Global Infobase 2010

| IASO | | | WHO GLOBAL INFOBASE | | |
|---|---|---|---|---|---|
| Country | Prevalence (%) | Rank (n=92) | Country | Prevalence (%) | Rank (n=192) |
| Nauru | 55.7 | 1st | Nauru | 84.6 | 1st |
| Tonga | 46.6 | 2nd | Cook Islands | 72.1 | 2nd |
| Cook Island | 40.6 | 3rd | Micronesia | 69.1 | 3rd |
| Kuwait | 36.4 | 4th | Tonga | 64.0 | 4th |
| French Polynesia | 36.3 | 5th | USA | 44.2 | 5th |
| USA | 35.5 | 6th | New Zealand | 28.9 | 15th |
| Canada | 27.6 | 11th | Australia | 28.4 | 16th |
| Scotland | 26.6 | 12th | Canada | 25.5 | 20th |
| England | 26.0 | 15th | UK | 23.7 | 23rd |
| Ireland | 25.8 | 16th | Ireland | 11.7 | 82nd |
| Australia | 25.6 | 17th | | | |
| New Zealand | 24.7 | 18th | | | |

*Source: IASO (2012) Prevalence data http://www.iaso.org/resources/. Accessed 2012. WHO Global Infobase International Comparisons https://apps.who.int/infobase/Comparisons.aspx? Accessed on 19/06/2013.*

**Table 2.4** Top five countries and selected other countries for obesity prevalence (BMI >30 kg/m$^2$) in females, IASO 2012 and WHO Global Infobase 2010

| IASO | | | WHO GLOBAL INFOBASE | | |
|---|---|---|---|---|---|
| Country | Prevalence (%) | Rank (n=141) | Country | Prevalence (%) | Rank (n=192) |
| Tonga | 46.6 | 1st | Nauru | 80.5 | 1st |
| Samoa | 63.0 | 2nd | Tonga | 78.1 | 2nd |
| Nauru | 60.5 | 3rd | Micronesia | 75.3 | 3rd |
| Kuwait | 47.9 | 4th | Cook Islands | 73.4 | 4th |
| Niue | 46.0 | 5th | USA | 48.3 | 13th |
| USA | 35.8 | 13th | New Zealand | 39.9 | 22nd |
| Scotland | 28.1 | 25th | Australia | 29.1 | 51st |
| England | 26.0 | 30th | UK | 26.3 | 56th |
| New Zealand | 26.0 | 30th | Canada | 25.7 | 61st |
| Australia | 24.0 | 35th | Ireland | 10.4 | 142nd |
| Canada | 23.5 | 41st | | | |
| Ireland | 25.8 | 51st | | | |

*Source: IASO (2012) Prevalence data http://www.iaso.org/resources/. Accessed 2012. WHO Global Infobase International Comparisons https://apps.who.int/infobase/Comparisons.aspx? Accessed on 19/06/2013.*

figures. The findings differ between organisations as the IASO reports straight figures from surveys that collect measured data within countries, whereas the WHO Global Infobase adjusts data to make it more comparable. This includes self-reported data.

Data presented by both organisations, however, suggest that Pacific Island populations have the highest obesity prevalence rates for adults throughout the world. Amongst developed countries the USA has the highest prevalence, ranked in the top ten for men by both organisations. The UK countries are also more highly ranked for men than for women.

## Child international prevalence

In addition to the difficulties of comparing between surveys collecting data in different countries at different times, comparing prevalence data for children is even more challenging due to the range of growth charts which are used internationally to determine weight status. Additionally surveys collecting data on children can collect from different age ranges making comparison even more difficult. The IASO compiles international figures on child obesity prevalence, presenting prevalence as determined by IOTF growth charts to allow comparison. They also provide details on the year of data collection and the age groups measured, so that informed comparisons can be made. From their figures the USA has the highest prevalence amongst developed and high-income countries (Table 2.5).

> ## ! Thinking points
>
> 1. Why is it useful to know prevalence data for other countries?
> 2. What are the weaknesses of using data that is modelled or adjusted?
> 3. What are the challenges in comparing between countries in obesity prevalence in adults?
> 4. What are the additional challenges in comparing child prevalence measurements?

## Adult international trends

Where data have been collected over a number of years by repeat cross-sectional surveys, trends in the prevalence of BMI status can be mapped. The Organisation for Economic Co-operation and Development (OECD) presents data over a number of years for 32 of its member countries. These data demonstrate large increases in the prevalence of obesity over the last 20 to 30 years for adults of both sexes (Figures 2.1 and 2.2). Similar trends have been found for children, demonstrating the increases in obesity over the preceding decades (see Box 2.1 and Figure 2.3). However, some question whether these prevalence rates are continuing to increase, with suggestions that for both adults and children they have slowed or even plateaued in recent years.[16] Others argue that it is too early to celebrate any kind

**Table 2.5** Obesity prevalence in children as determined by IOTF growth charts, age range and year of survey, IASO 2011

|                  | BOYS (%) | GIRLS (%) | YEAR OF SURVEY | AGE RANGE (YEARS) |
|------------------|----------|-----------|----------------|-------------------|
| Australia        | 22.0     | 24.0      | 2007           | 2–16              |
| Canada           | 28.9     | 26.1      | 2004           | 6–17              |
| England          | 22.7     | 26.6      | 2007           | 5–17              |
| New Zealand      | 28.2     | 28.8      | 2007           | 5–14              |
| Northern Ireland | 27.0     | 25.0      | 2005           | 2–15              |
| USA              | 35.0     | 35.9      | 2003/4         | 6–17              |

*Source: IASO (2012) Prevalence data http://www.iaso.org/resources/. Accessed 2012.*

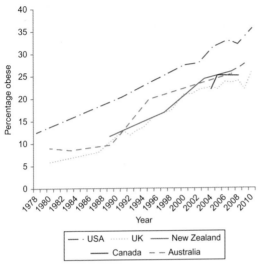

**Fig. 2.1** *Percentage of obese men in selected countries, OECD, 1978 to 2009. Source: Based on data from OECD Health Data (2012). Obesity, percentage of male population with a BMI>30 kg/m², based on measures of height and weight. OECD Frequently requested dataset, accessed on 23/1/2012.*

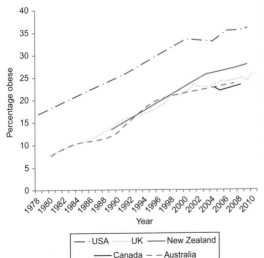

**Fig. 2.2** *Percentage of obese women in selected countries, OECD, 1978 to 2009. Source: Based on data from OECD Health Data (2012). Obesity, percentage of female population with a BMI>30 kg/m², based on measures of height and weight. OECD Frequently requested dataset, accessed on 23/1/2012.*

**Box 2.1 Case study: Childhood obesity trends in England**

Health Survey for England (HSE) data suggest a plateauing in the prevalence of childhood obesity since 2005.[2,17] However, these data also show some relationship to sample size, which differs across recent years of data collection. When investigating the absolute difference of obesity prevalence between each data collection and the year with the largest sample size (2007) for the last seven data collections, there is some suggestion of the prevalence converging as the sample size increases (Figure 2.3). A similar relationship is found for overweight and obesity prevalence and mean BMI. Recent peaks in prevalence, found in 2004 and 2005, also coincide with the smallest sample sizes. This could lead to less confidence in the prevalence measures for years in which data collection was from smaller samples which might not be picked up when simply reporting trends, or in statistical testing that investigates a trend across many years.[18] Knowledge of the data is, therefore, important before any conclusion is drawn from statistical tests. Deciding whether the sample is typical of the population is not a statistical issue, but rather will depend on an informed judgement using knowledge of the biology and epidemiology of the population.[19]

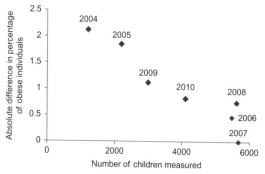

**Fig. 2.3** *Absolute difference in obesity prevalence to largest sample size in children aged 2–15 years, Health Survey for England 2004 to 2010.*
*Source: Townsend et al. (2012) Evaluating the evidence that the prevalence of childhood overweight is plateauing. Paediatric Obesity; 2012; 7(5): 343–6.*

of levelling off in prevalence, adding the difficulties in the comparative data collections between years mean that we need many years of figures before we can be confident that any change in the direction of trends is occurring. It is certainly clear that annual fluctuations do occur in prevalence figures from surveys, reflecting differences in data collection rather than genuine annual changes in prevalence. Due to the nature of obesity it is unlikely that genuine meaningful changes will happen over the course of 12 months. Trends need to be judged over a longer period of time in order to determine any directional change.[17] What all authors agree on is that irrespective of the direction of recent trends current prevalence figures are too high in almost all high-income countries.

## Predicting future trends

Predicting future trends in the prevalence of obesity on a national and international level is difficult, as many assumptions must be made in order to predict how obesity prevalence will change, whilst not being able to control for unknown future events. Additionally much of the outcome is dependent on the data that are being used, such that should surveys show particular trends due to issues other than population

prevalence changes, such as data collection issues which are not obvious, these could influence the predicted trend.

The 2007 Foresight Report *Tackling Obesities: Future Choices* by the UK Department of Health included a micro-simulation model that works at the level of the individual to attempt to predict future trends for a number of scenarios in the UK, up to the year 2050.[20] Within this report these estimations suggested alarming rises in prevalence over the next four decades (Table 2.6) for all ages.

In 2011 Wang et al. used the same approach with more recent prevalence data to predict future trends up till 2010 for a number of countries.[21] In doing so they predicted increases for a number of countries (Figure 2.4).

The OECD also undertook a modelling exercise to project trends in adult overweight and obesity for ages 15–74 years of age for OECD countries

**Table 2.6** Measured prevalence in 2007 and modelled estimates for prevalence in 2050 in England, by age and sex

| AGE | MALES (%) | | FEMALES (%) | |
|---|---|---|---|---|
| | 2007 | 2050 | 2007 | 2050 |
| 1–20 (IOTF) | 7 | 26 | 10 | 26 |
| 21–30 | 15 | 42 | 13 | 30 |
| 31–40 | 28 | 65 | 22 | 47 |
| 41–50 | 26 | 55 | 23 | 52 |
| 51–60 | 32 | 65 | 27 | 49 |
| 61–70 | 31 | 64 | 32 | 59 |
| 71–80 | 28 | 63 | 27 | 44 |

*Source: Butland, B. et al., 2007. Tackling obesities: future choices – project report (2nd edn), London: Foresight Programme of the Government Office for Science.*

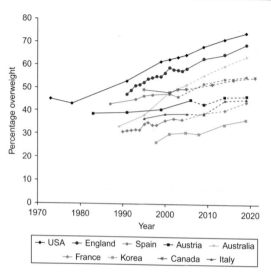

**Fig. 2.4** *Modelled estimates of adult obesity prevalence in selected countries, 1970–2020. Source:[21] Health and economic burden of the projected obesity trends in the USA and the UK. The Lancet; 378 (9793):815–825.*

up until 2020, by extrapolating past trends, thereby assuming that the entire distribution of BMI in national populations would continue to evolve following the patterns observed in the past. In doing so they assume that the factors that have determined these increases in prevalence over recent years, including approaches adopted by governments to tackle increases, will continue to exert the same influence on future trends. They reported projections which suggest a continued increase in obesity rates in OECD countries, with these increases greater in countries in which prevalence has historically been lower, such as France and Korea.

**Thinking points**

1. What must be considered in following a trend over years using data from surveys or measurement programmes?
2. What are the difficulties in attempting to predict future prevalence figures and trends?
3. How many years of data collection must be collected if we are to determine a trend in prevalence?
4. Why should predicted increases in prevalence be greater for countries with lower current prevalence figures?

# Prevalence within countries

As well as differences between countries in prevalence figures, it is also common to find differences in prevalence between subgroups of the national population within countries. These are not always easy to determine, however, as stratifying data by a number of factors reduces the number of individuals from which data were collected, leading to problems of small samples. There are a number of characteristics by which prevalence figures can differ within a national population.

## Sex

In many high-income countries obesity prevalence is similar between the sexes, with some small differences, but amongst men a higher prevalence of overweight and obesity is often found. However, male and female adults are judged by the same BMI cut-offs which may not take account of the greater mean muscle mass found in men. Indeed using the BMI and waist circumference WHO classification which has different waist circumference cut-offs for men and women, a greater percentage of women in England are found to be at high risk or very high risk compared with men. Amongst children for whom different growth charts are used for the sexes, boys are found to have a higher prevalence of obesity than girls in most high-income countries. Opposing relations are found in some countries in which women are found to have a higher prevalence of obesity, such as Tonga and Samoa.

## Age

Differences in the prevalence of weight status can also be found by age in both adults and children. In most countries data suggest that older children are at a greater risk of obesity than younger children and the prevalence of obesity amongst adults increases with age up until late middle age. There is a slight decrease in obesity prevalence into older age. Figures 2.5 and 2.6 demonstrate this relationship in English data, but similar findings are apparent in most developed countries. There are difficulties in comparing older children to younger adults as BMI status is defined by growth charts in children and by a standard BMI threshold in adults of all ages.

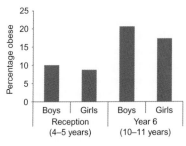

**Fig. 2.5** *Percentage of obese children by sex and school year group in England, NCMP, 2010/11. Source: National Health Service Information Service 2012. National Childhood Measurement Programme, England, school year 2010/11.*

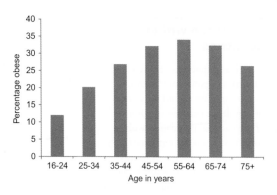

**Fig. 2.6** *Percentage of obese adults in England by age in years, Health Survey for England, 2010. Source: Health Survey for England 2010 Copyright © 2012, Re-used with the permission of The Health and Social Care Information Centre. All rights reserved.*

## Ethnicity

Inequalities in obesity risk related to ethnicity have been identified in a number of countries.[22–32]

The 2009–2010 NHANES found differences between ethnic groups in prevalence of obesity amongst adults[33] as well as ethnic differences between children, with non-Hispanic white children less likely to be obese than Hispanic children (including Mexican Americans) and non-Hispanic black children. They also reported differences in trends between 1999 and 2010 between ethnic groups.[9]

In Australia, comparing data from the 2004–2005 National Aboriginal and Torres Strait Islander Health Survey (NATSIHS) to the 2004–2005 National Health Survey (NHS), after adjusting for differences in the age structure of the two populations, indigenous men were 1.6 times as likely to be obese and indigenous women were more than twice as likely (2.2) as non-indigenous women. The 2008/9 New Zealand Health Survey found that Pacific Islanders had a higher prevalence of obesity for both men (56.2%) and women (59.5%) than Maoris (men 40.7%, women 48.1%) and those of European origin (men 24.8%, women 23.7%).

Differences are also apparent between ethnic groups amongst children in England with data from the NCMP suggesting that the Black ethnic groups had the highest prevalence of obesity and Chinese the lowest. However, these results should be treated with caution as they are only based on the BMI method, and the definitions of overweight and obesity in the UK are taken from growth charts compiled using data from White children only. The NCMP also suggests that developments in the changes in both height and BMI across ages are different between ethnic groups. This leads to a further complication as there is a suggestion that BMI may be correlated with height amongst children, such that taller children are more likely to be classified as overweight.[34,35] Although there is also evidence that obese children may be taller younger than the non-obese, these findings come from studies that either focus on one ethnic group[36] or have stratified findings by ethnic group[37] and do not compare between them. Additionally, research using dual-emission X-ray absorptiometry (DXA) and triceps skinfold thickness, suggests that children in Black ethnic groups, who tend to be taller in childhood,[38,39] carry less fat for the same level of BMI than other ethnic groups, whilst South Asians tend to carry more.[39]

These differences in body composition are also a challenge in comparing between ethnic groups amongst adults. Data from England found many differences between ethnic groups in obesity prevalence with these relationships differing depending on the type of measurement. Although Black African and Black Caribbean ethnic groups had a higher prevalence of obesity amongst men, as determined by BMI, compared to South Asian ethnic groups, this was reversed when classifying risk by waist/hip circumference ratio measurements (Figure 2.7). However, different relationships are found between ethnic groups amongst women (Figure 2.8).

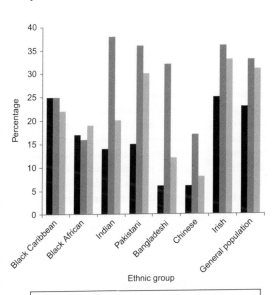

**Fig. 2.7** *Body mass index, waist-hip ratio and waist circumference by ethnic group, men, 2004, England. Source: Health Survey for England 2004 Copyright © 2012, Re-used with the permission of The Health and Social Care Information Centre. All rights reserved.*

■ BMI of 30 kg/m² and over ■ Waist-hip ratio 0.95 and over
■ Waist circumference 102 cm and over

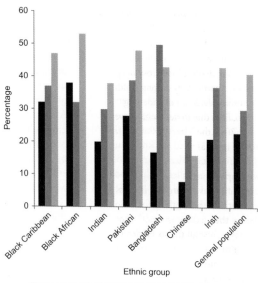

**Fig. 2.8** *Body mass index, waist-hip ratio and waist circumference by ethnic group, women, 2004, England. Source: Health Survey for England 2004 Copyright © 2012, Re-used with the permission of The Health and Social Care Information Centre. All rights reserved.*

Difficulties can also occur in the collection of data. To be comparable data must be collected from large numbers of individuals in each ethnic group. This is difficult for minority ethnic groups (MEGs) due to low numbers in the population. Often to overcome a lack of power in sample sizes, some studies have been stratified by large age ranges[24,40,41] or grouped MEGs that might not be homogeneous in obesity risk into larger groups such as 'Asian',[23,40] 'South Asian',[39,42,43] 'Indo-Pakistani',[41] 'Indian Subcontinent',[44] 'Pakistani and Bangladeshi'[45,46] and 'Black'.[47] The definition of ethnicity can also prove a challenge in determining differences between groups. Ethnicity can include a number of dimensions which may imply shared origins, social background, culture and traditions,[48] with this concept made more complex due to migration and the mixing of ethnic groups.[49] Although it proves very difficult to create mutually exclusive categories of ethnicity[50] it is often treated as a fixed characteristic, with this definition of ethnicity often self-defined in data collection.[51]

## Deprivation

There is much evidence linking deprivation to adiposity,[52] although this relationship can vary by characteristics such as age, sex and ethnicity.[53,54] In England, as in other developed countries, obesity is associated with social and economic deprivation across all age ranges,[55] particularly among children,[56,57] with some evidence of widening inequalities due to deprivation over time.[56]

In 2010 the Marmot Review into health inequalities in England *Fair Society, Healthy Lives* emphasised the importance of reducing health inequalities as a matter of fairness and social justice, calling for action to reduce the gradient in health, not only obesity, across all the social determinants of health.[55] The review recommends a community focus to tackling these inequalities as the physical and social characteristics of the area in which an individual lives make a contribution to social inequalities,[55] as well as to the development of overweight and obesity,[58] with evidence that area-level deprivation is associated with obesity independently of individual SES.[58] Within *Fair Society, Healthy Lives*, proportionate universalism is promoted, in which actions are determined with a scale and intensity proportionate to the level of disadvantage within communities.[55]

Age-standardised HSE data by household income equivalised by the number of individuals in the house shows no significant differences in mean waist circumference by income in men. However, in women, mean waist circumference was highest for those in the lowest income quintile (90.6 cm)

and lowest in those in the highest income quintile (85.0 cm). Similarly, the prevalence of raised waist circumference was highest among women in the lowest quintile (52%) and lowest in women in the highest quintile of income (36%) (Figure 2.9).

Among children aged 2–15, there was variation both in mean BMI and in the proportion of children who were obese according to equivalised household income. Mean BMI was lowest among girls living in households in the highest income quintile (17.5 kg/m$^2$), and increased as equivalised income decreased (19.3 kg/m$^2$ in the lowest quintile), although there was no similar variation among boys. Reflecting the pattern with mean BMI, girls in the highest two income quintiles were the least likely to be obese (6% in the highest quintile and 8% in the second highest), and those in the lowest two quintiles were the most likely (19% and 21%). The pattern was slightly different among boys, with similar proportions obese in the highest four quintiles, and a higher proportion in the lowest quintile (20%) (Figure 2.10).

Data from the NCMP demonstrate an increase in obesity prevalence for both girls and boys with increasing deprivation of the place of residence. With research suggesting that this relationship holds for deprivation at the area and school level and that the effect of deprivation is greater for older children.[59]

**Fig. 2.9** *Prevalence of obesity and raised waist circumference by quintile of equivalised household income for adults in England, by sex, 2010. Source: Health Survey for England 2010 Copyright © 2012, Re-used with the permission of The Health and Social Care Information Centre. All rights reserved.*

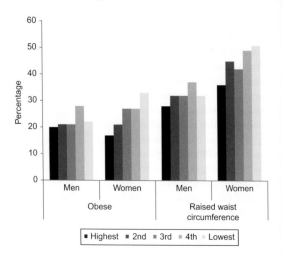

**Fig. 2.10** *Prevalence of obesity and raised waist circumference by quintile of equivalised household income for children in England, by sex, 2010. Source: Health Survey for England 2010 Copyright © 2012, Re-used with the permission of The Health and Social Care Information Centre. All rights reserved.*

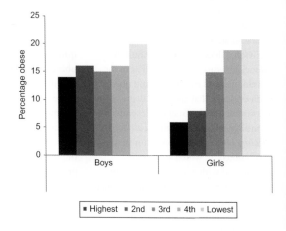

The New Zealand Adult Nutrition Survey shows a trend in increasing prevalence with increasing deprivation in women varying from 16.5% obese in the quintile with the lowest deprivation to 41.2% in the quintile with the highest deprivation. Any trend is less clear amongst men although the most deprived quintile also has the highest prevalence (33.4%); the lowest prevalence is found in the middle quintile (23.7%).

Data from NHANES found that among men, obesity prevalence is generally similar at all income levels, with a tendency to be slightly higher at higher income levels according to poverty income ratio. Although this differed by ethnic group, a stronger trend was shown amongst women, for whom prevalence of obesity increased with increasing poverty. However, increases in obesity were found between 1988–1994 and 2007–2008 for all income levels.[60]

NHANES data also found that among both boys and girls, obesity prevalence decreases as income increases, but this relation is not consistent across race and ethnicity groups. Children and adolescents living in households where the head of household has a college degree are less likely to be obese compared with those living in households where the household head has less education, but the relationship is not consistent across race and ethnicity groups. Between 1988–1994 and 2007–2008 the prevalence of childhood obesity increased at all income and education levels.[60]

## Regions

Geographic inequalities in health in a number of countries are strong. In England regional differences in overweight and obesity prevalence mirror those of other disease and risk factors, with higher levels in the North than in the South, particularly for women. In the last 10 years the gap between women in the South of England and the North of England has increased.[61] Regional and geographical differences in prevalence are reported by the HSE and the NCMP, which collects rich enough data to produce prevalence estimates at small regional separation. Regional differences are also presented by a number of other national surveys, although this requires collecting data from a large enough number of individuals from every region to present prevalence figures with confidence. Comparing between regions can be misleading, however, as differences between regions in demographics such as age, ethnicity and deprivation may be shaping differences in prevalence (see Figure 2.11).

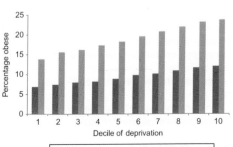

**Figure 2.11** *Prevalence of obesity by decile of quintile of Index of Multiple Deprivation of area of residence for children in England, 2010. Source: Joint Health Surveys Unit, 2012. National Child Measurement Programme 2011/12. The Information Centre: Leeds. Copyright (C) 2012, Re-used with the permission of The Health and Social Care Information Centre. All rights reserved.*

## ! Thinking points

1. What are the weaknesses of using the same BMI cut-offs for men and women?
2. What are the challenges in comparing between subgroups of the population, such as ethnic groups, in prevalence?
3. What can be done to make regions more comparable in prevalence despite differences in demographic make-up?
4. What are the challenges in collecting prevalence figures for minority ethnic groups?

## Summary points

- Cross-sectional surveys or measurement programmes allow for the estimation of national prevalence figures of obesity, with much of these data available online.
- The most recent survey data from the UK suggest over one quarter of adults are obese, compared to more than one third in the USA.
- More than half of all adults in the countries discussed in this chapter are overweight or obese, with this as high as two thirds in some countries.
- Over one quarter of children in the UK, USA and Australasia are overweight or obese, although prevalence differed between countries and by sex, and were calculated using different growth charts.
- A number of organisations compile international data on obesity and make them available online for comparison.
- To make prevalence comparable some organisations adjust or model collected measurements.
- Using IOTF growth charts, over one third of children in the USA are obese, whilst over one fifth are in England and Australasia.
- The Pacific Islands are found to have the highest prevalence in adult obesity among countries in the world.
- Repeat cross-sectional surveys or measurements programmes allow us to follow trends in prevalence over time.
- Surveys suggest dramatic increases in prevalence of obesity in both adults and children over the preceding three decades. Extrapolating recent trends and micro-simulation modelling suggest prevalence will continue to rise.
- Although some authors point towards recent levelling off in prevalence in recent years, it is too early for a confident conclusion to be made and these trends may be influenced by data collection.
- In the UK, North America and Australasia a higher prevalence of men than women are overweight or obese.
- Prevalence of obesity increases with increasing age until older age groups in adults.
- Differences are found between ethnic groups for all obesity measures in many countries.
- Individuals living in more deprived areas or who are poorer are more likely to be obese.

## Web pages and resources

British Heart Foundation (BHF) Heart statistics website.
www.bhf.org.uk/research/statistics.aspx.
International Association for the Study of Obesity (IASO).
www.iaso.org/.
The World Health Organisation (WHO) Global Infobase.
https://apps.who.int/infobase/.
The WHO Global Database on Body Mass Index.http://apps.who.int/bmi/index.jsp.

## Further reading

1. Finuacane, et al. National, regional, and global trends in body-mass index since 1980: systematic analysis of health examination surveys and epidemiological studies with 960 country-years and 9.1 million participants. Lancet 2011;377(9765):557–67.
*This paper written by members of the Global Burden of Metabolic Risk Factors of Chronic Diseases Collaborating Group describes trends in BMI from 1980 to 2008 on a global, national and regional level.*

2. Olds, et al. Evidence that the prevalence of childhood overweight is plateauing: data from nine countries. Paediatr Obes 2011;6:342–60.
*The authors present data from nine countries which suggest childhood obesity is levelling off.*

3. Townsend, et al. Evaluating the evidence that the prevalence of childhood overweight is plateauing. Paediatr Obes 2012;, Epub 2012.
*The authors provide a commentary on the Olds et al. paper discussing evidence suggesting a decrease in childhood obesity; in doing so they discuss issues that should be considered when evaluating evidence from measurement programmes and surveys.*

# 3 The health consequences of obesity

Being overweight or obese can increase the risk of developing a range of chronic diseases, with these risks rising with increasing BMI.[1] This has led some to compare obesity to smoking in terms of its associated disease burden and as a determinant of future health.[2,3] As well as a link to morbidity of disease BMI has also been found to be a strong predictor of mortality amongst adults, with being obese found to reduce life expectancy by over five years.[4]

The effects of obesity on the body include the physical changes that occur due to the increased mass of fatty tissue as well as changes at the cellular and metabolic levels. These physical changes lead to difficulties such as musculoskeletal problems which arise due to increased mass as well as psychological and social challenges caused by altered body image and stigma. Many of the effects of overweight and obesity, however, arise due to the increased production of various substances by the fat cells and an altered response to insulin.

The direct impact of obesity on health is not always clear, however, as evaluating the health consequences of excess adiposity can prove difficult.

## Difficulties evaluating the health consequences of obesity

The World Health Organization (WHO) identify five specific problems in evaluating the health consequences of obesity:[5]

1. Overweight and obesity are defined at particular thresholds of BMI; however, there is a continuous relationship between BMI and both morbidity and mortality, and weight gain in individuals will not always cause individuals to change BMI status.
2. Health behaviours may impact on both BMI and health, leading to erroneous conclusions on the impact of BMI on health.
3. It is difficult to develop a study that will allow a focused investigation

into the link between BMI and health outcomes. Illnesses such as cancer develop after many years and as result of multiple factors, of which BMI is one. Long-term longitudinal studies which collect data on a number of measures are therefore required for a focused investigation.

4. The age of participants in studies is also important; studying older individuals allows for the study of mortality, whereas BMI at a young age is an important predictor of future cardiovascular disease.

5. Initial BMI is commonly used in studies, but weight gain is seen as an important risk factor with the type of fat gained also key. Measuring both of these in a large enough number of people to develop confident findings is very challenging.

> **Box 3.1 Common abnormalities associated with intra-abdominal fat accumulation**
>
> - Increases in leptin, adiponection and resistin
> - Increased insulin resistance and increased insulin secretion
> - Abnormalities in the balance of sex steroids
> - Increased free testosterone and free androstenedione levels associated with decreased sex hormone binding globulin (SHBG) in women
> - Decreased progesterone in women
> - Decreased testosterone in men
> - Increased cortisol production
> - Decreased growth hormone levels
> - Increased concentrations in the inflammatory cytokines
>
> *Sources:*[5–7,9–11]

## Fat as an active tissue

Besides its role in storing energy in the form of lipids, adipose tissue is a metabolically active endocrine organ[6] with the adipocytes acting as endocrine cells by releasing and receiving hormones. This can lead to changes in hormonal patterns[7] especially amongst those with abdominal fat.[8] The substances the adipocytes release are called adipocytokines and they are associated with a range of systemic or local actions including glucose and lipid metabolism, cell development, CVD, cancers, metabolic conditions including diabetes, inflammation, oxidative stress and the metabolism of sex steroids.[7] These substances released by the adipocytes along with the changes in hormonal balance lead to a number of the health problems described throughout this chapter (Box 3.1).

## Abdominal fat

Although the risk of suffering obesity-related ill health has been found to increase with increasing BMI, the type of fat an individual is carrying is an important factor. General fat accumulated in the lower body below the waist is subcutaneous, as it lies between the skin and the muscle. Fat found around the abdomen can be either subcutaneous or it can be visceral. Visceral fat lies underneath the muscle and surrounds the abdominal organs. Fat can also be found behind the abdominal cavity when it is referred to as retroperitoneal fat, although this is generally considered to be visceral fat.

Several studies indicate that visceral fat is more strongly correlated with ill health than subcutaneous fat. Visceral fat has a higher density of cells, carries more blood flow, and more receptors for hormones whilst research suggests that the visceral fat cells are also more biologically active, producing hormones and other substances, such as cytokines. Additionally visceral fat is located close to the portal vein which carries blood from the intestine to the liver. This results in increases in the amounts of fatty acids which reach the liver[12] affecting the production of blood lipids. An association has been found between visceral fat and higher levels of total cholesterol, in particular low-density cholesterol (LDL), also leading to lower concentrations of high-density cholesterol (HDL).

## Types of ill health associated with obesity

Excess adiposity is associated with a large range of health consequences related to the following:

- Circulatory system.
- Cancer.
- Metabolic.
- Gastrointestinal and liver.
- Musculoskeletal.
- Respiratory system.
- Reproductive health.
- Urology.
- Psychological and social difficulties.
- Dermatology.

## Circulatory system

### Hypertension
One of the most profound effects of obesity on the circulatory system is its link to hypertension, which is itself a risk factor for a range of CVDs. Both systolic and diastolic blood pressure have been found to increase with increasing BMI, with an estimated 65% to 75%

---

### ! Thinking points

1. How can excess adiposity and the behaviours that lead to it be separated in studies so that the independent effect of obesity on ill health is identified?
2. What types of studies are best suited to investigate the impact of obesity on health?
3. How do smoking and obesity compare as risk factors for ill health?
4. What makes visceral fat a greater risk factor than subcutaneous fat?

of hypertension risk attributed to excess weight.[3,13] Obese individuals are therefore more likely to be hypertensive with the risk of hypertension found to increase with an increasing duration of obesity.[14]

## Elevated cholesterol

Obesity has an effect on the metabolism of lipoproteins, with increasing weight found to lead to increases in the concentrations of triglycerides and low-density cholesterol (LDL). Obesity has also been found to be linked to decreases in the concentration of high-density cholesterol (HDL) with this relationship found to be greater for abdominal fat.[14] Obese individuals are therefore at a greater risk of dyslipidemia than non-obese individuals.[3,14]

## CVDs

Obesity promotes clusters of risk factors that greatly increase CVD risk (Box 3.2) including accelerated coronary atherosclerosis,[16] hypertension, dyslipidaemia, insulin resistance, increased coagulability, endothelial dysfunction, and inflammation.[17-22] This places obese individuals at a substantially elevated risk of CVDs such as heart failure,[23] peripheral vascular disease,[24] deep vein thrombosis and pulmonary embolism.[3,14,25] The obese have also been found to have an increased risk of stroke with three of the key risk factors (hypertension, CHD and diabetes) directly related to obesity.[3] Evidence suggests there is a stronger link

---

**Box 3.2 Case study: The Framingham Heart Study**

The Framingham Heart Study is a long-term, on-going longitudinal study on cardiovascular disease, recruiting participants from the town of Framingham, in Massachusetts, USA. The study began in 1948 with 5209 adult subjects aged 30 to 62 years of age at initial examination. It is currently in its third generation of participants.[15]

Participants were followed for up to 44 years to study changes in risk factor status with a number of cardiovascular disease end points monitored. The overall results from the study indicated that these CVD outcomes were highly associated with obesity. Calculating population attributable risks (PAR) for these conditions allowed researchers to estimate the reduction in incidence of a number of CVDs in the population if none of the participants in the Framingham Heart Study had been overweight or obese.

The CVDs most highly associated with overweight and obesity included angina pectoris (PARs=26% in men and 22% in women) and total CHD (PARs=23% in men and 15% in women) with results for total CVD similar to these (PARs=16% in men and 17% in women). They also reported associations between overweight and obesity and CVD risk factors such as hypertension (PARs=26% in men and 28% in women), hypercholesterolaemia (PARs=10% in men and 9% in women) and diabetes (PARs=21% in men and 3% in women).[15]

between stroke and waist-to-hip ratio than BMI,[26] indicating the importance of abdominal obesity in this risk.

Recent evidence, suggests, however, that as well as promoting risk factors for CVD, obesity has also been found to be an independent risk factor for both CHD morbidity and mortality. CHD risk is more acute in younger age groups[22] and higher in relation to those with abdominal obesity.[27]

## Cancer

The International Agency for Research on Cancer has reported that individuals who are overweight or obese are at increased risk of developing several types of cancer. It has also been reported that conditions associated with obesity, including hyperinsulinaemia and hormonal changes, increase the risk of cancer.[28] The increased incidence of hormone-dependent cancers is found to be more prominent for those with abdominal adipose, which is thought to have a direct link to hormonal changes.

Calle and Kaaks (2004) presented relative risks and population attributable fractions (PAFs) for both the US and European Union populations, describing increased risk for many cancers for both the overweight and the obese as determined by BMI (Table 3.1).

Although the link to breast cancer among premenopausal women is less

**Table 3.1** Increased risk of different cancers for overweight and obese with PAFs for US and EU populations

| TYPE OF CANCER | RELATIVE RISK FOR BMI 25–30 kg/m² | RELATIVE RISK FOR ≥30 kg/m² | PAF (%) FOR US POPULATION | PAF (%) FOR EU POPULATION |
|---|---|---|---|---|
| **Hormone dependent** | | | | |
| Endometrial | 2.0 | 3.5 | 56.8 | 45.2 |
| Breast (postmeno-pausal women) | 1.3 | 1.5 | 22.6 | 16.7 |
| **Gastrointestinal/hepatic/renal** | | | | |
| Colorectal (men) | 1.5 | 2.0 | 35.4 | 27.5 |
| Colorectal (women) | 1.2 | 1.5 | 20.8 | 14.2 |
| Gallbladder | 1.5 | 2.0 | 35.5 | 27.1 |
| Pancreatic | 1.3 | 1.7 | 26.9 | 19.3 |
| Liver | Not determined | 1.5–4.0 | Not determined | Not determined |
| Renal | 1.5 | 2.5 | 42.5 | 31.1 |
| Gastric cardia | 1.5 | 2.0 | 35.5 | 27.1 |
| Oesophageal | 2.0 | 3.0 | 52.4 | 42.7 |

Source: Calle and Kaaks (2004). Nature reviews. Cancer, 4 (8), pp. 579–591.

strong than found for postmenopausal women[29] there also appears to be an important link between obesity and breast cancer in men, with reports that obesity may double the risk of developing the disease.[30] Breast cancer in men is much less common than in women, however, and as such does not constitute as large a public health concern.[3]

Other hormonal cancers that have been linked to obesity include prostate cancer, for which there is evidence of a small increased risk for all forms of prostate cancers,[28] and large increases in the risk in developing more severe types such as metastatic disease.[31] There is also an increased risk of ultimately dying from the disease.[32,33] Cancer of the thyroid has been found to be associated with increasing BMI, with this relationship stronger amongst men.[34] Premenopausal ovarian cancer is associated with a high BMI measured in women at 18 years of age.[3,35]

There is also some evidence of obesity increasing the risk of developing blood cancers such as multiple myeloma[3,28,36,37] and non-Hodgkin lymphoma.[3,38–41]

# Metabolic

## Diabetes

The risk of type 2 diabetes, also known as non-insulin-dependent diabetes mellitus (NIDDM) is substantially raised with higher BMI,[42] with one estimate suggesting that a 20 kg weight gain leads to a 15-fold increased risk of diabetes.[43] There are a number of characteristics associated with obesity that have been reported to increase the risk of type 2 diabetes; these include obesity in childhood and adolescence as well as progressive weight gain from 18 years of age. Intra-abdominal fat has also been found to be an independent risk factor for diabetes[44] which is also associated with increased risk of pre-diabetic conditions including impaired glucose intolerance and insulin resistance. The risk of diabetes is also associated with the severity and duration of obesity.[3,43]

## Metabolic syndrome

Metabolic syndrome describes the clustering of a number of CVD risk factors which are associated with obesity. These include abdominal obesity, impaired glucose intolerance, elevated blood pressure, high LDL/low HDL and insulin resistance.[45] The combination of these abnormalities has been shown to be highly predictive of end-point diseases such as coronary artery disease, stroke and diabetes.[45]

Each component of metabolic syndrome increases the CVD risk independently, but together they interact to increase risk synergistically. This concept of a clustering of risk factors was first described in the 1920s, whilst a link to obesity was first made in the 1940s.[45] Although it is commonly referred to as the metabolic syndrome, it is also referred to as syndrome X, the insulin resistance syndrome and the deadly quartet.[45]

The ultimate importance of metabolic syndrome is that it helps identify individuals at high risk of both type 2 diabetes and cardiovascular disease (CVD).[46] It can, however, be hard to diagnose in individuals as it can present in various ways according to the different components that make it up.[42] Although there have been a number of guidelines which can be used to diagnose metabolic syndrome,[46] here we present those from the International Diabetes Federation who published guidelines in 2006. This uses an obesity classification, or ethnic-specific waist circumference measure, along with two out of four other conditions to determine a diagnosis of metabolic syndrome (Box 3.3 and Table 3.2).

# Gastrointestinal and liver

## Gallstones

Obesity has been found to be a risk factor for gallstones in all ages and both sexes, with this association stronger for those with abdominal adiposity. Overweight and obesity are linked to supersaturation of bile with cholesterol, the primary material in gallstones,[47] along with

---

**Box 3.3 International Diabetes Federation: metabolic syndrome definition**

To be defined as suffering from metabolic syndrome patients must have a BMI ≥ 30 or ethnic-specific central obesity as defined by waist circumference (see Table 3.2) plus any two of the following conditions:

1. Raised triglycerides:
   >150 mg/dL (1.7 mmol/L)
   Specific treatment for this lipid abnormality
2. Reduced HDL-cholesterol
   <40 mg/dL (1.03 mmol/L) in men
   <50 mg/dL (1.29 mmol/L) in women
   Specific treatment for this lipid abnormality
3. Raised blood pressure
   Systolic ≥130 mmHg
   Diastolic ≥85 mmHg
   Treatment of previously diagnosed hypertension
4. Raised fasting plasma glucose
   Fasting plasma glucose ≥100 mg/dL (5.6 mmol/L)
   Previously diagnosed type 2 diabetes
   If above 5.6 mmol/L or 100 mg/dL, oral glucose tolerance test is strongly
      recommended, but is not necessary to define presence of syndrome.

*Source: Alberti et al. (2006) Diabetic Medicine: A Journal of the British Diabetic Association, 23 (5), pp. 469–480.*

**Table 3.2** Ethnic specific central obesity for metabolic syndrome definition

| ETHNIC GROUP | | WAIST CIRCUMFERENCE (cm) |
|---|---|---|
| Europids | | |
| | Men | ≥94 |
| | Women | ≥80 |
| South Asians | | |
| | Men | ≥90 |
| | Women | ≥80 |
| Chinese | | |
| | Men | ≥90 |
| | Women | ≥80 |
| Japanese | | |
| | Men | ≥85 |
| | Women | ≥90 |
| Ethnic and south central Americans | | Refer to South Asians recommendations until more specific data available |
| Sub-Saharan Africans | | Refer to Europids recommendations until more specific data available |
| Eastern Mediterranean and Middle East (Arab) populations | | Refer to Europids recommendations until more specific data available |

Source: Alberti et al. (2006) Diabetic Medicine: A Journal of the British Diabetic Association, 23 (5), pp. 469–480.

reduced motility of the gallbladder; both of these are factors for the formation of gallstones. These can lead to gallbladder inflammation which is also more common in obese individuals.[48] Obese individuals have a higher risk of requiring gallbladder surgery.[49]

## Pancreatitis

Pancreatitis (inflammation of the pancreas) caused by activation of digestive enzymes in the pancreas is strongly associated with both dyslipidaemia[3,50,51] and gallstones, which are more common in the obese. Obesity has been found to be associated with an increased risk of pancreatitis and increased severity and likelihood of developing complications.[3,52–54]

## Gastroesophageal reflux disease (GERD)

Gastroesophageal reflux disease (GERD) also known as GORD, gastric reflux disease, or acid reflux disease, is caused by stomach acid coming up into the oesophagus. An increasing risk of GERD has been found with increasing BMI,[48,55] which has also been linked with more severe GERD[56] with this association stronger for women than men.[57] One of the links between obesity and GERD may be an increased risk of hiatal hernia in the obese, meaning that the diaphragm cannot act as a barrier to stop acid leaking into the oesophagus.[3,57] The increased intra-abominal pressure caused by the accumulation of intra-abdominal fat, along with the higher incidence of abnormal contractions of the oesophagus in the obese, may also be a factor.[3,58,59]

### Non-alcoholic liver disease

Adipose tissue, and in particular visceral fat, is a primary factor in the development of non-alcoholic fatty liver disease (NAFLD). Accumulation of fat in the liver is mostly dependent on recirculating free fatty acids (FFAs) from adipose tissue. The release of these fatty acids directly into the portal vein by visceral fat is an important mechanism in this.[60]

Other gastrointestinal conditions are associated with obesity, and may arise due to other gastric conditions associated with excess adiposity. These include: upper abdominal pain, potentially caused by physical distention of the stomach after episodes of eating or delayed gastric emptying; diarrhoea, potentially caused by the increased amount of food consumed; chest pain/heartburn; vomiting; retching and incomplete evacuation.[48,55]

## Musculoskeletal

### Joint pain

Raised body weight puts strain on the body's muscles and joints which can lead to the development of a number of conditions, as well as joint pain. An association has been found between increasing BMI and the symptoms and severity of joint pain.[61] Increasing BMI, specifically abdominal fat, is also strongly associated with foot pain and disability.[62] In obese persons, pain is most prevalent in the load-bearing joints, including the lower limbs particularly the knee and the lower back.[63,64] Excess adiposity can lead to impairment of the spine[65,66] and has been recognised as being a risk factor for chronic lower back pain. However, it can also manifest in upper extremity joints including the hands and digits,[67] the thoracic spine, and the neck.[61] From a biomechanical perspective obesity induces abnormal joint loads and leads to adverse changes in the composition, structure, and properties of articular cartilage. When strength is normalised for body mass, obese individuals are found to have lower muscle strength than their normal-weight counterparts.[68,69] Within obese individuals, skeletal muscle becomes laden with intramuscular fat which releases biomarkers that lead to muscle breakdown and further loss of strength.[61,70] On many occasions obese individuals attempt to compensate for muscle weakness and instability by altering gait patterns and adopting different body transfer patterns to move excessive weight.[61]

### Osteoarthritis

In many instances joint pain may reflect the underlying pathologic process of osteoarthritis (OA) which itself is associated with obesity. For every 5 kg of weight gain, a 36% increased risk of developing OA has been reported.[61,71] With inadequate lower limb strength in obese individuals, there is less absorption of the impact forces on weight-bearing joints and joint misalignment may occur.[61] Repetitive forces then damage the articular cartilage, leading to OA.[61,72] Additionally, excessive adipose tissue compresses load-bearing joints and creates an inflammatory environment, whilst skeletal muscle becomes laden with intramuscular fat, both of which contribute to the onset of osteoarthritis.[61,70] Inflammation is also mediated by the activities of several adipokines which are released by adipose tissue, with recent evidence suggesting that some of these contribute to cartilage breakdown.[61,73]

### Gout

Gout is a highly prevalent form of inflammatory arthritis.[74] The increased risk of gout for obese individuals is thought to be related to the accompanying hyperuricaemia (increased uric acid levels) as well as increased mass. There is some suggestion that excess abdominal fat may lead to a greater risk of gout.[75]

### Other musculoskeletal conditions

There is evidence that obese individuals suffer deficiency in vitamin D,[76,77] possibly because vitamin D is fat-soluble, so adipose tissue may store the vitamin, making it unavailable to the rest of the body.[76] Vitamin D is essential for absorption of calcium, so a lack of the vitamin can lead to a weakening of the bones and associated conditions. However, there is some evidence that osteoporosis may be less common amongst the obese,[78,79] which could be due to increases in mechanical load strengthening the bones.[80] However, evidence suggests that excess body fat may be linked to lower bone mass once the effects of mechanical loading are accounted for.[3,81]

## Respiratory system

### Respiratory function

Obesity is associated with alterations in a number of respiratory functions. Alterations to the respiratory mechanics including airway resistance, changes to the pattern and work of breathing, and reductions in lung capacity all lead to decreased gas exchange and lower levels of oxygen available to the body.[82,83] These changes in function are thought to be due to the increased elastic load posed by excess weight on the thorax and abdomen,[3,84] increased pulmonary blood volume and ventilation–perfusion mismatch.[82]

## Male fertility

BMI also affects male fertility, with reductions in fertility occurring at a BMI greater than $35 \, kg/m^2$. Studies have shown impairment of fertility, or sperm count, associated with massive obesity, with the relationships between reduced sperm concentration and BMI exhibiting a clear dose–response relationship.[109–111] The risk of oligospermia (sperm concentration <20 million sperm/mL) has also been found to be higher in overweight and obese men than in normal weight individuals, with a similar relationship found with obesity as determined by BMI and waist-to-hip ratio.[112,113] This may in part be explained by decreased testosterone production, hypogonadotropism[114] and increased testicular temperature[111,115] due to extra skin, excess body fat and enlargement of the veins in the scrotum.[116] Partners of obese men have also been found to be less likely to conceive[3,117,118] especially if the partner themselves is obese.[117]

## Erectile dysfunction

Both an increased risk of erectile dysfunction and reduced coital frequency have been found to be associated with obesity[119,120] in part due to decreased testosterone production and production of adipocytes.[111,121] Associated CVD symptoms may also have an effect[122,123] including affecting the blood vessels of the penis.[3,124]

## Contraceptive failure

Contraceptives which use hormones to affect pregnancy such as oral contraceptives, implants and transdermal patches have all been found to be less reliable in obese women.[125–127]

## Pregnancy

Obesity has been found to link to maternal complications during pregnancy including hypertensive disorders, diabetes, infection, thromboembolism, altered mood, and complications during labour and delivery, such as foetal distress, arrest of active phase of labour and dystocia (including shoulder), abnormal presentation, with obese women requiring increased rate of instrumental delivery and caesarean section.[128–130] Obesity can also impair the use of some technologies, such as ultrasound scans used to detect abnormalities in the foetus.[131] Obesity increases the risk of operative delivery and complications including impaired recovery.[132] Prematurity is strongly associated with obese mothers, mostly related to induction of labour and caesarean section from pre-eclampsia.[133] The risk of foetal death is also greater with increasing BMI and is not restricted to early pregnancy[134,135] with recurrent miscarriage associated with obesity[99,135] and hyperinsulinemia.[136,137] Obesity is linked to an increased risk of foetal abnormalities,[135,138] whilst the associated mortality of the child is not in a negative light and believe others wish to exclude them from social life.[12]

## Depression

Bidirectional associations have been found between obesity and depression[155] and anxiety disorders.[156] Studies describe a link between severe obesity and greater risk of depression[157,158] whilst it has also been found that extremely obese people who seek bariatric surgery have lower self-esteem and higher depression scores than less obese individuals who seek pharmacological and behavioural weight loss interventions.[159] Many patients are depressed about their condition and the negative impacts of obesity.[160] There is also evidence that people with chronic or repeated episodes of depression are at particular risk of subsequent obesity.[161] Research has found that women experience greater dissatisfaction with their weight and shape than men do, and this dissatisfaction increases with increasing BMI.[162]

## Dementia

Adiposity in mid-life is associated with an increased risk of dementia in old age, independent of sociodemographic characteristics and common comorbidities[163,164] with midlife obesity linked to an increased risk of developing both Alzheimer disease and vascular dementia.[165] The link with dementia is unclear although CVD and diabetes, both associated with obesity, have also been found to link to dementia.[166,167] A link between adipocytines and dementia has also been suggested.[3,163,168]

## Dermatology

### Skin infections

Obese individuals are more prone to skin infections such as those that occur in skin folds; due to friction, warmth and moisture, as they have a greater number of folds which are deeper leading to more sweat production and more moisture.[24,169] Associated conditions such as CVD and diabetes also increase the risk of these.[24] These skin infections include intertrigo in which the top layers of the skin are infected with fungus or bacteria, as well as infections of the deeper layers of the skin such as infectious cellulitis, gas gangrene and necrotising fasciitis, all of which are associated with obesity, diabetes and impaired circulation.[3,24,169]

### Acanthosis nigricans

Acanthosis nigricans, a condition of darkening and roughening of localised areas of skin including on the arms, the back of the neck, scalp and knees is more common amongst the obese and is also associated with diabetes.[169]

### Psoriasis

It has been suggested that psoriasis is more common amongst obese individuals.[170] Although there is no evidence of causation, some obesity-related diseases such as NALD or hypertension may interfere with treatment for the condition.[3,171]

## Pressure sores

Pressure sores can develop in obese patients due to poor blood supply to the adipose tissue[169] and due to pressure where skin folds touch. This is particularly the case where obese individuals are using equipment such as chairs or beds which are not suitable for their size, or where patients are immobile.[3]

## Stretch marks

Stretch marks in obese individuals occur due to the pressure on the skin from expanding body fat[43] leading to stretching and thinning of the connective tissue.[169]

---

**!** **Thinking points**

1. Are there certain conditions associated with obesity which should be targeted above others?
2. Which of the measurements discussed in Chapter 1 best identifies those individuals at a greater risk of obesity-related ill health?
3. Which conditions have a bidirectional association with obesity?
4. All of the conditions included in metabolic syndrome are related to ill health, why is it so important to identify when they are present as a part of this syndrome?

---

# Differences in risk between ethnic group

The relationship between obesity-related ill health and BMI is not the same for all individuals with important differences in risk found between ethnic groups.[172] These risks of ill health vary by generation of migration and can partially be explained by factors associated with ethnicity such as socioeconomic factors.[173–175] A higher prevalence of obesity-related diseases in minority ethnic groups (MEG) than in the white population in USA has been reported, with this particularly the case for NIDDM, CVD and stroke, whilst osteoarthritis is also found to be more common in Black Americans.[176] In the UK the risks of CVD have been found to be greater at lower BMI in many South Asian groups.[177] An elevated risk of hypertension has been found amongst South Asians even when BMI is low, whilst mortality rates for CHD are higher for first-generation migrants to England.[172] Individuals from South Asian ethnic groups have been found to be at a greater risk of diabetes and other metabolic syndromes[178] whilst obesity-related psychosocial problems also differ between ethnic groups. Black females in America and the UK have been found to experience less social pressure about their weight[179] and to have higher self-esteem.[180] However, US-born black women, along with US-born non-Hispanic white women, have been found to be more likely to suffer obesity-related depression[181] with health status a mitigating factor.[181] South Asians who are obese have been found to be at particular risk of low self-esteem.[180,182]

## Children and adolescents

The most significant long-term impact of childhood obesity is its persistence into adulthood with this more likely in late childhood and when obesity is severe.[183,184] Overweight and obesity in adolescence have been found to be significantly associated with adult mortality and morbidity.[185]

There are a number of psychological and social difficulties associated with obesity[3,186,187] with these emotional and psychological effects of being overweight often seen as the most immediate and most serious by children themselves. They include teasing and discrimination by peers; low self-esteem; anxiety and depression.[188,189]

Conditions which are particular to children include an early timing of puberty[190,191] which can lead to psychological problems and reproductive cancers.[190] Conditions of the musculoskeletal system including Blount's disease, a severe bowing of the legs due to overgrowth of the tibia caused by extra weight; spinal complications;[192] hip problems and slipped capital femoral epiphysis (SCFE),[193] which can require surgical correction.[194] Pseudotumour cerebri, characterised by increased pressure from the cerebrospinal fluid that surrounds the brain, which can lead to vision impairment, is more common amongst the obese, although causality is unproven.[186]

## Mortality

Due to the increased risk of ill health, obesity is associated with shorter life expectancy. In 1987 Bray described a linear or curvilinear relationship between obesity and mortality, beginning at a BMI of around 20 to 22. A number of more recent studies have attempted to quantify the link between BMI and mortality and have produced similar results. The Prospective Studies Collaboration meta-analysis (2009) described the lowest mortality in the BMI range 22.5 to 25 kg/m$^2$ and an increase of 30% overall mortality for every 5 kg/m$^2$ increase in BMI above the discovered optimum of 22.5 kg/m$^2$.[195] This meant individuals within the 30 to 35 kg/m$^2$ range had a life expectancy reduced by two to four years and those in the 40 to 50 kg/m$^2$ range by eight to ten years.[195] The Framingham Heart Study suggested that obesity at the age of 40 led to a decrease in life expectancy of around six years in males and around seven years in females.[4] It is paradoxical, therefore, that at a time when obesity rates are at their highest, life expectancy is increasing in many countries. This increase can be explained by decreases in some diseases, particularly CVD, due to improvements in treatments and associated decreases in risk factors, especially smoking. Some authors argue that mortality statistics based on obesity as the underlying cause alone may substantially underestimate obesity-related deaths.[196]

> ⚠ **Thinking points**
>
> 1. How can we account for differences between ethnic groups in obesity-related ill health?
> 2. Are there additional factors which should be considered when investigating obesity-related ill health in one MEG?
> 3. Obesity in any individual is of concern; why is it especially so in children?
> 4. What is the danger of seeing one BMI value as the optimum for life expectancy?

## Societal impact of obesity

As well as the individual impact of obesity-related ill health, there is also a societal impact. Studies from both the USA and UK have predicted an overall decrease in life expectancy.[197,198] Although some have argued this will not be too great in some cases,[199] others have suggested that this has been alleviated to some degree by decreases in other risk factors such as smoking.[200] Much research, however, suggests that the impact of obesity on disability is far larger than its impact on mortality[201] as the obese develop chronic disease earlier and live more of their lives with these diseases[202] including diabetes, hypertension and OA.[203] Disability, as defined as a limitation in the ability to perform activities of daily living (ADL), is much greater in the obese.[204,205]

## Economic impact of obesity

There are also financial impacts of obesity-related ill health accrued both through treatment costs, with one review suggesting that obese individuals were found to have medical costs 30% greater than their normal weight peers,[206] but also through the loss of earnings as ill health or early death removes individuals from the work force.

A review in the USA found that the direct medical costs per individuals are $266 higher for obese individuals, and the incremental costs $1723 higher, than that of normal-weight persons, leading to an aggregate national cost of overweight and obesity of $113.9 billion.[207] It has been suggested that Medicare and Medicaid finance approximately half of these obesity-related medical costs.[208] Similar results have been found in other countries with an estimated $21 billion annual total direct cost of overweight and obesity reported in Australia in 2005.[209] Direct costs to the UK NHS from obesity and related ill health have been estimated to be as high as £4.2 billion[199] with much of this cost through treating obesity-related type 2 diabetes and hypertension.[210] Costs have also been accrued in purchasing specialist equipment for larger individuals, including large-sized beds, chairs, operating tables, radiological equipment and hoists.[211] The combined annual medical costs associated with treatment of these obesity-related diseases are estimated to increase by as much as $66 billion in the USA and by £2billion in the UK by 2030[212] with costs to the UK NHS predicted to rise to £9.7 billion by 2050.[199]

The costs of obesity on society do not stop with treatment costs, as indirect costs are also accrued in relation to earnings lost due to premature mortality and obesity-related ill health and disability. In 2004 a House of Commons Health Committee (HCHC) estimated total costs of obesity to the UK to be between £3.34 billion and £3.72 billion.[213] A later assessment in the Foresight report in 2007 estimated indirect total costs of obesity in England to be around £15.8 billion.[214] The direct and indirect costs of obesity and obesity-related illnesses in Australia in 2008/09 were estimated to be $37.7 billion; this included $6.4 billion lost due to lost productivity arising from absenteeism, presenteeism and premature death.[215] The total annual economic costs associated with obesity in the USA are estimated to be in excess of $215 billion.[216] A report by the Society of Actuaries estimated that total annual economic cost of overweight and obesity in the United States and Canada caused by medical costs, excess mortality and disability is approximately $300 billion.[217]

---

### Thinking points

1. Why is it important to consider the societal and economic impacts of obesity?
2. Which should be considered more in formulating treatments for conditions such as obesity, the societal or the economic impacts?
3. Do the considerations of countries related to the direct costs of treating obesity differ depending on the type of health service they have?
4. How would countries increase revenue to cover the total costs of obesity and what impact would this have on other aspects of society?

---

### Summary points

- There are several challenges to measuring the impact of obesity on health.
- The behaviours that lead to obesity are also associated with ill health.
- Fat is an active tissue, releasing several substances and hormones.
- Visceral fat is more closely linked to ill health as it is more active and releases fat into the blood.
- Obesity is related to a huge range of conditions within the body.
- Metabolic syndrome is important as it highlights individuals at an elevated risk from a number of conditions.
- The link between obesity and ill health can occur due to both increased mass and substances released by the fat cells.

*Continued*

- As well as physical ill health, obesity is associated with a range of psychological and social difficulties.
- There are inequalities in obesity-related ill health found between ethnic groups.
- Childhood obesity also incurs a number of risks, the most important of which is continuation of obesity into adulthood.
- Overweight and obesity are associated with higher mortality, and with decreases in life expectancy found with increasing BMI.
- The optimum BMI in relation to mortality has been found to be around $22.5\,kg/m^2$.
- The decreased life expectancy and increased disability associated with obesity lead to impacts on society.
- Costs to health services include direct costs of treating obesity and treating obesity-related ill health.
- Costs to the economy are accrued through loss of work days through disability and death.
- These costs are predicted to rise in many countries.

## Web pages and resources

National Obesity Observatory. Obesity and Health.
www.noo.org.uk/NOO_about_obesity/obesity_and_health.

Endocrine function in obesity.
http://www.sciencedirect.com/science/article/pii/S2173509311000250.

Harvard School of Public Health. The Obesity Prevention Source Economic Costs.
www.hsph.harvard.edu/obesity-prevention-source/obesity-consequences/economic/.

CDC. Obesity.
www.cdc.gov/chronicdisease/resources/publications/aag/obesity.htm.

## Further reading

1. Kava, et al. Obesity and its Health Effects. New York: American Council on Science and Health; 2008.
   *This report published by the American Council on Science and Health presents an extensive summary of the impact of obesity on ill health.*
2. Sassi F. Obesity and the Economics of Prevention: Fit Not Fat. OECD Publishing; 2010.
   *This publication discusses health and societal impacts of obesity including economic impacts and the economics of prevention.*
3. Berenson G. Health consequences of obesity. Pediatr Blood Cancer 2012;58:117–21.
   *This paper presents findings from the Bogalusa Heart Study of the association between obesity in childhood and adult and CVD outcomes.*

* To view the full reference list for the book, click here http://dx.doi.org/10.1016/B978-0-7020-4634-6.09992-1

# 4 **Causes of obesity**

Weight gain in terms of an increase in adipose tissue in the body comes as a result of an energy imbalance, where energy taken in has been greater than energy used over a period of time.[1] If we consider the first law of thermodynamics, which states that 'energy cannot be created or destroyed; it can only be changed from one form to another' we recognise that when energy taken in, in the form of food and drink, exceeds that expended through homeostasis or physical activity, the excess energy will be converted into another form: adipose tissue.[2] Although the relative importance of energy intake and expenditure may vary between individuals, and at different stages of life, when we describe population increases in obesity, these come about due to an overall population increase in positive energy balance.[3]

This relatively simple concept of energy balance can hide the complex nature of the behaviours that lead to energy intake and expenditure and the large number of interactive influences on these.[4] In an attempt to demonstrate the complex nature of the determination of obesity the UK Government Office for Sciences published an obesity system map as a part of its Foresight report.[2] This map, which many recognise as the most comprehensive compilation of the determinants of obesity and their inter-relations,[5] consists of 108 variables and 305 causal linkages.

## Energy balance

### Energy intake
Energy intake is determined by the type and quantity of food eaten, with different types of food containing different amounts of energy. In considering the main food categories: fat, protein, carbohydrate, fibre and alcohol, we find that fat has the highest energy density and so delivers more energy through the diet than other foods (Table 4.1). It is readily stored as body fat with minimal energy costs and proves to be less satiating than

**Table 4.1** Energy content of macronutrients

| MACRONUTRIENT | ENERGY CONTRIBUTION | |
| --- | --- | --- |
| | kcal/g | kJ/g |
| Fat | 9 | 37 |
| Alcohol | 7 | 29 |
| Protein | 4 | 17 |
| Carbohydrate | 4 | 16 |
| Fibre | 1.5 | 6 |

Source: WHO (2000) Preventing and Managing the Global Epidemic.

other food groups,[6] with fatty foods also thought to encourage overeating (passive overconsumption).[7]

Fibre, in comparison, limits energy intake by lowering food density and allowing time for appetite control signals to occur before large amounts have been consumed. This can lead to incomplete digestion and energy absorption[7] and greater satiation due to the increased demands on chewing and digestion.[8,9] Fruit and vegetables are examples of food that tend to have low energy density and are high in fibre.[10] Although there is some evidence that protein may act as a satiety cue,[11] in general, there is little evidence of any special role for protein in appetite control.[12,13]

Energy consumed in liquid form appears to supplement habitual food intake rather than replace it. This can then lead to increases in body weight,[14–16] in particular with consumption of sugary soft drinks[17] which may displace more nutritious fluids in the diets of young children.[18]

Diets characterised by food high in fat or sugar and relatively low in fibre have been associated with greater weight gain[19–21] with diets which include a large proportion of energy-dense processed foods linked to an increase risk of obesity.[22–24] Although overall energy balance is the most important factor in weight control it must also be noted that diet influences health independently to body weight.[25,26]

# Regulation of energy intake

Long-term regulation of energy balance can be influenced by adipose tissue itself, which has a direct role in regulating appetite through feedback loops involving the release of hormones such as leptin, leading to a mechanism to produce an equilibrium in fat levels over a period of time.[27] A drop in the concentration of leptin initiates hunger, whilst increases lead to feelings of satiety.[28]

The more short-term regulation of energy intake, through food, at any one time is also under the control of a number of feedback loops. Levels of hormones such as ghrelin, which is released when the stomach is empty, generate hunger, with these decreasing as the stomach fills. When enough food has been eaten stretch receptors in the stomach wall send nerve messages to the brain and hormones such as cholecystokinin are produced by the digestive system to generate feelings of fullness. These responses are not immediate, however, and it is estimated to take around twenty minutes for stretch receptors and hormones to tell the body that it is satiated.[29,30] This means that individuals cannot rely solely on feelings of hunger and satiation to monitor how much to eat and they must learn to determine portion size through experience.

Some refer to an asymmetry of appetite in which individuals respond to the efficient hunger signals to eat, but the inefficient satiety signals do not work so quickly to suppress appetite, when the individual has eaten enough or when they do not require a lot of energy.[31] Additionally, in high-income countries where there is a surplus of energy-dense, low-cost food, this metabolic control is easily overcome[28,30,32] by sensory factors such as sight, smell and palatability which interact with availability to promote appetite. This is commonly known as 'hedonic' hunger.[30]

## Energy expenditure

The energy expenditure of an individual is determined by their basal metabolic rate (BMR), adaptive thermogenesis and the energy expended through physical activity.[33,34] BMR refers to the numerous biochemical processes needed to sustain life that occur constantly within the human body. Adaptive thermogenesis is the energy used in the form of heat in response to environmental change, whereas physical activity describes all voluntary movement by an individual.[34]

Although the amounts of energy required by these three processes vary between individuals, BMR makes up the primary component accounting for between 60 and 70% of total energy expenditure. It is important to recognise that there is little evidence to support the belief that obese people have lower metabolic rates than the non-obese. Controlled studies reveal that slim and obese individuals show similar rates of weight gain and loss when over- or under-fed.[35,36] Indeed energy requirements actually increase as individuals gain weight, as metabolic requirements of the individual increase due to the increased mass, along with the additional cost of activity at this heavier weight.[1,37,38] This can lead to a dynamic phase in which weight is put on, being followed by a static phase in which weight is maintained at a higher level of energy requirements.[1,37,38]

Adaptive thermogenesis, resulting from heat loss, diet and other factors accounts for around 10 to 15% of total energy requirement and can vary due to lifestyle, whereas physical activity accounts for the remaining energy requirement.[39] Physical activity shows the most variation between individuals and is the volitional component. It has been found that physical activity can contribute as little as 5% or as much as 30% of total energy expenditure for different individuals[40] with the types of physical activity also found to vary between individuals of different ages and sexes.[41,42]

Physical activity therefore proves to be a critical component of energy balance as it can account for the differences in fat storage that occur in individuals who are overfed[43] allowing individuals to avoid weight gain. A well-established inverse relationship is found between BMI and physical activity,[44,45] with a greater risk of being overweight or obese associated with increased sedentary behaviour.[25] There is also evidence that increases in weight can increase sedentary behaviour[46–48] with large individuals finding it difficult to be active. Additionally, the energy consumed during active exercise also leads to increases in BMR due to the replenishing of energy supplies, including those in the form of glycogen found in the liver and muscles, along with the increases in respiring tissue in the form of muscle mass.[46,48]

As with diet, physical activity influences health independent of body weight and is of benefit to all individuals and not just the obese.[25,26]

> **! Thinking points**
>
> 1. Why does the formation of obesity have so many interacting factors?
> 2. Is there a time at which the asymmetry of appetite could have proved advantageous?
> 3. What factors can override the biological control of appetite and satiety?
> 4. Why is physical activity the form of energy expenditure which varies the most between individuals?

## Influences on obesity

The high current population prevalence of obesity has arisen as a result of a genetic and biological suitability for an environment in which food was scarcer and higher levels of activity were required, interacting with a modern environment in which food is plentiful for many and lifestyle has become more sedentary. Genes that may have conferred an evolutionary advantage to gorge and store fat in times of food excess are now less suitable in the current environment that were first described as obesogenic in the 1990s. Obesogenic refers to the sum of the influences that promote obesity[49] which is the net result of biological, behavioural, and environmental impacts acting through the mediators of energy intake and expenditure.[50] These produce effects over a number of years and throughout the life course of an individual.[4,51]

# Individual influences on obesity

## Biological/genes

Studies have suggested that some individuals are more susceptible to becoming overweight and obese than others due to biological and genetic factors.[1] Genetic research has led to a suggested multi-gene effect, with over 250 genes, markers or chromosomal regions identified that may potentially influence body weight.[52] It has been suggested that genetics can explain 25–40% of the individual difference in adipose tissue.[53] However, although there is evidence that a number of specific genes are associated with excess adiposity[54–56] these genes commonly interact with the environment to do so.[1,2] It is rare that genes directly cause overweight or obesity, whilst the rate of increase in obesity prevalence in populations is greater than could be expected from genetic changes, pointing to environmental change as the main driver.[1,2] The developing study of epigenetics takes this relationship further as it describes not only interactions between genes and the environment to develop a phenotype, but also the impact of the environment on the expression of genes themselves.[57] Although an individual knowledge of genetic susceptibility may lead to a targeting of interventions, it is still likely to lead to suggestions to influence energy intake in a way which can be achieved without a knowledge of individual genetic makeup.[2] In fact if we are to reverse the increasing trend in obesity we must 'cure' the environment which has led to these increases rather than target the genes with which the environment has interacted.[58]

## Sex

Obesity prevalence is generally higher in females than males and differences are also found between the sexes in the distribution of fat within the body. These sex differences arise due to hormonal differences influencing body composition and appetite along with behavioural, socio-cultural and chromosomal factors.[59]

Although there is some evidence of preferential storage of fat amongst females, men are found to be at an increased risk of obesity-related ill health because they are more likely to develop visceral fat than premenopausal women, due to hormonal differences.[59]

In general men appear to be more active, whilst women are more likely to follow a healthy diet, respond to health messages,[60] value health more and adopt preventive strategies.[61] Women have lower energy expenditure on average than men for height and weight due to lower mean muscle mass and have been found to benefit less from physical activity due to differences in metabolic responses. They have also been found to be more likely to increase energy intake after exercise to account for this increased expenditure.[59]

Sex differences also occur through different social pressures around thinness with research suggesting that body image and emotional factors play a more significant role in the development and maintenance of obesity in women, with differences found between the sexes in the way that they respond to stress.[59]

### Age

The influences that encourage obesity vary across the life course, with those at an early age thought to be particularly important, not least as obesity in childhood is likely to persist into adulthood.

Intra-uterine nutrition,[62] birth weight[63,64] and breastfeeding[65] have all been found to be linked to adult body weight, with recent studies also suggesting that infants delivered by caesarean section may be at increased risk of childhood obesity due to physiological differences in the infant.[66] A poor maternal diet during pregnancy is a risk factor for low birth weight, which in turn has been associated with abdominal obesity in adulthood.[67] The relationship between birth weight and BMI in childhood and young adulthood is often thought to be linear with those of a lower birth weight found to have proportionately more adipose tissue and a greater proportion of this being centrally located.[68] More recent evidence suggests it may be J or U shaped, indicating an increased risk at heavy and light extremes.[69]

Being breastfed has been associated with a reduced risk of obesity in childhood and adolescent overweight.[70–72] Findings for this are inconsistent[73] or suggest a small effect,[74] although it has been found that exclusive breastfeeding for several months offers best protection.[72]

Rapid and early weight gain in infancy is associated with an increase in the risk of obesity,[75] as is the early introduction of complementary foods (before 16 weeks of age).[76]

Adolescence is a key time for weight gain, as it is associated with autonomy and a change of food and physical activity habits, as well as some physiological developments, in particular in puberty[77,78] during which overweight individuals gain significantly more weight than those who are normal-weight.[79]

There are more changes to diet and physical activity patterns both on entering adulthood and throughout it. These are commonly influenced by lifestyle changes which occur throughout the life course. These include marriage, the birth of a child or changes in employment.[80–83] Giving up sport or an active hobby can lead to fat gain, due to decreases in physical activity and the loss of muscle tissue[84] if these changes are not compensated for by decreasing energy intake.

Pregnancy is also a significant factor in encouraging weight gain in women[85–87] as are the lifestyle changes after pregnancy.[88] Postpartum weight gain has been associated with increased food intake, greater access to food during the day, lower levels of exercise, increased time watching television, and less social support.[89] Although breastfeeding can account for an extra energy loss in new mothers[90] as there is an energy cost for milk production,[91] most women follow a pattern of partial breastfeeding, which is not associated with substantial weight loss[86] with the strongest influence on weight retention thought to be the amount of weight gained during pregnancy.[87]

Hormonal changes that occur throughout adulthood also impact on weight gain. In men, the observed gradual decline in circulating androgens, often referred to as 'andropause' is accompanied by increased total and abdominal fat and decreases in muscle mass, which occur in part due to reductions in circulating hormones.[92] Menopause is a high-risk time for weight gain in women.[59,93] Although there is some suggestion that age and lifestyle could be the main causes for weight gain at this time, it has also been found that menopause is associated with an increase in abdominal fat independent of age and total body fat.[94] Hormone replacement therapy (HRT) which at one point was considered to increase body weight, is now thought to have little impact and may even reduce abdominal fat.[95–97]

## Socioeconomic status

Socioeconomic status (SES) (a measure of an individual's or family's social position relative to others) is linked to adiposity,[98] with those from lower SES backgrounds in high-income countries found to indulge in more obesogenic behaviours, such as eating more energy-dense food and being less physically active.[99] This relationship is found to be stronger for women than men[100] and is also true for children,[101] with SES in childhood a predictor of obesity in adulthood. However, there is some evidence that women are more likely to adopt the BMI standard of the SES they move to later in life.[102] The relationship between SES and obesity can vary by characteristics such as age, sex and ethnicity[103,104] with an opposing relationship found in many lower-income countries where obesity can be considered a sign of affluence and lead to less healthy dietary behaviour.[105]

Some have suggested it is economic inequality which accounts for most of the social inequality in obesity rates,[106] with the price elasticity of various foods decreasing with increasing income,[107] so that as consumers become more affluent they respond less to price changes in food. The cost of food may thus be one barrier to adopting healthier diets, with studies suggesting that energy-dense and nutrient-poor foods provide dietary energy at lower cost than do more healthy foods.[108,109] Additionally less affluent individuals are more concerned by food waste and are therefore less likely to buy foods that will be wasted, leading to more restricted diets.[110] Although the economics prove to be important they are not the only factor. There are links between SES and environmental influences, including likelihood of breastfeeding,[111–114] nutrition in infancy and childhood, psychological factors and cultural or social norms in relation to diet choice and attitudes to body shape.[102] Some studies also report a reverse causality between SES and obesity, in that obesity adversely affects SES. It is possible, however, that external factors may influence both SES and obesity simultaneously.[115,116]

## Ethnicity

The prevalence of obesity has been found to vary between ethnic groups, with it commonly greater for minority ethnic groups (MEGs) due in part to differences in both physical activity and dietary choice.

Low levels of physical activity have been found for MEGs[117,118] with greater sex disparity.[119] This is also true amongst children where some MEGs have been found to be less active and demonstrate faster rates of decline in activity in adolescence.[120,121] Some MEGs view an incompatibility between sport and femininity[122] including culturally specific demands in relation to dress codes, modesty and the need for single-sex facilities[119] and the need for culturally appropriate exercise facilities.[123]

Differences in diet have also been found between ethnic groups[124] with evidence that many MEGs are engaged in poor dietary behaviour.[125] Cultural practices and knowledge about food preparation have been found to influence this.[126,127] The fast aspect of cuisine is most likely to be integrated into the eating habits of immigrants as the price of familiar food products and a lack of availability, along with long preparation time can drive them away from traditional dishes.[128] Younger ages and younger generations are more likely to change their diet to processed foods[129] highlighting the link between migration and obesity.[130–132]

Additionally, although the Western cultural preference for slenderness has been adopted by many minority ethnic communities, younger generations in pursuit of this can feel constrained by the opinions of older generations' cultural attitudes in favouring larger body sizes.[128,133,134] On occasions this conflict can lead to a 'layering' of stigma where Western and MEGs stigmas clash.[135]

The independent influence of ethnicity is not always clear, however, as individuals from MEGs are more likely to be of low SES and live in poverty[136–139] and are spatially concentrated in deprived urbanised areas.[140] However, a buffer of social support has been found in areas with large numbers of the same MEGs.[141,142]

> **! Thinking points**
>
> 1. Can a focus on genetic links to obesity help us counter it on a population level?
> 2. Why are the early life influences on obesity so important in comparison with others that occur later in the life course?
> 3. What factors could create a bidirectional relationship between BMI and SES?
> 4. What influences might change between generations in the same ethnic groups?

### Intrapersonal

Intrapersonal factors deal with those that reside within a person, within the self or mind, such as personality and attitudes towards health behaviours. These include food preferences, eating patterns and habits, beliefs, knowledge and self-efficacy.

Food preference is an important factor in food choice and tends to promote consumption, with fat and sugar often leading to more palatable foods.[143] Preference would appear to have some genetic determination,[144] although it is also strongly influenced by the environment, with all individuals born with a neophobia towards eating certain foods, which is overcome through influence from carers.[145,146] There is also a psychological conflict between lifestyle desire and the desire to be healthy or slim, which complicates individual choices.[147]

Unhealthy foods are often seen as desirable whilst it can be difficult to find time to be active in the modern lifestyle.[148]

Knowledge or beliefs towards healthy behaviours are also important in shaping health outcomes. However, although knowledge provides individuals with the ability to know how to make healthy choices[149,150] it is clear that nutritional knowledge alone does not significantly influence food behaviour; knowing how to eat healthily does not necessarily mean individuals will do so.[151] Individual beliefs are also an important influence, with differences found between individuals as to whether the degree of positive outcomes or the creation of less negative ones is more important.[2] Additionally there is evidence that emotional factors are at odds and dominant over material or factual information.[2] Ambivalent individuals tend to respond to health promotion messages in a polarised fashion, either extremely positively or extremely negatively. They also scrutinise messages and may form negative attitudes to messages if they are flawed or too simplistic.[147,148,152]

Self-efficacy (belief that the individual is capable of performing a behaviour)[153] is found to be a predictor of success in weight loss,[154] weight management[155] and healthy dietary choice.[156,157] There is evidence that self-efficacy can be enhanced with therapy.[158]

Habits (repeat behaviours triggered by cues and decoupled from the original reason for behaviour) can be difficult to overcome.[147] Individuals who have developed habits are less likely to respond positively to new messages and change behaviour.[2] Such habitual behaviours are characterised by 'tunnel vision' in which the individual does not wish to use information to understand the impact of their behaviour, or discounts new information received, particularly when it suggests risks for this habit.[4]

Stress has been found to have a bidirectional relationship with obesity. There is some evidence of a biological link between stress and body weight with cortisol, the hormone released at times of stress, associated with the development of visceral and abdominal fat.[159,160] It has also been found to link to appetite regulators such as leptin,[161,162] although this is not consistent with all individuals.[163–166]

Changes in other behaviours can also lead to weight gain. For example giving up smoking is associated with an increase in weight[167–169] although this can be attenuated by levels of physical activity, age, baseline BMI and the rate of smoking.[169] Weight control is, therefore, important for individuals who are giving up smoking and should not be discouraged due to the increased risk from smoking over obesity.[170] Alcohol intake is also associated with abdominal fat[171] as are certain prescription drugs.[172–176] Holidays can also lead to behaviour change that is associated with changes in body weight.[177,178]

## Interpersonal

Interpersonal factors are concerned with an individual's social environment and involve relationships between individuals. These influences can affect eating behaviours through mechanisms such as modelling, reinforcement, social support, and perceived norms.[179,180] These mechanisms act through the social interactions of individuals within the primary groups with whom they socialise; these primary groups include family, friends and peer networks. Identifying interpersonal influences can be difficult, however, as these individuals commonly share the environment in which they live.[181–184]

Parental obesity is a risk factor for obesity in offspring, with a higher likelihood for children to be overweight or obese if at least one of their parents is.[4] BMI in childhood is strongly related to maternal BMI.[185] Parents' reported fruit and veg intake has been found to be the strongest predictor of children's intake[186] as parents' food preferences influence those of their children through role modelling and choice in the availability of food.[187]

There is some evidence that infants initially adjust food intake in response to energy requirements, but with age they lose this individual regulation and become increasingly reliant on external stimuli.[10] As parents provide environments for their children's experiences with food and physical activity they significantly influence their children's behaviours.[188,189]

Parental presence at meal time is associated with a lower risk of poor consumption of fruits, vegetables and dairy food, and the likelihood of skipping breakfast,[190] which can lead to overconsumption and unhealthy snacking later in the day.[191,192] Parents can play a role in shaping dietary patterns which are linked to obesity, including meal frequency, consumption of food from outside the home, beverage consumption, portion sizes, and dietary quality.[188] A high frequency of family meals is associated with a healthy diet and lower consumption of unhealthy foods and in particular a reduction in the number of ready-made dinners consumed.[193]

Several studies have shown that parents who use inappropriate techniques to try to control and modify their children's eating behaviour may actually promote the development of unhealthy eating styles and childhood overweight.[194] Restricting foods can lead them to be desirable, particularly if they are known to be available, and using unhealthy foods as a reward can make them more appealing.[195]

Peer pressure, social convention and religious practices can all lead to determining behaviours related to obesity.[4,196] A link has been found between individual weight and friends' and family weight gain.[4,196] Adolescent weight is correlated with that of individuals of the same age in the peer group.[4,197,198] Whilst spousal weight can also be linked, spouse choice may influence this.[4,199]

The celebration of festivals is often associated with particular foods and can lead to weight gain[200,201] with this worse for individuals with a higher BMI at baseline for whom this gain is less likely to be reversed.[200,201]

---

> ### Thinking points
>
> 1. Why is knowing how to eat healthily not enough to encourage healthy eating?
> 2. Why is it important that individuals are born with a degree of neophobia?
> 3. How do those individuals who influence us change as we age?
> 4. How can rewarding children with unhealthy food in order to encourage them to eat healthy food create undesirable eating behaviours?

---

## Environmental factors

Although obesity has a range of causes, the environment is the key factor in its rapid rise. Dietary patterns in most high-income countries are thought to have changed, mostly as a result of rising incomes and an increasing food supply, which some refer to as the nutrition transition.[202,203] The availability of fast food has increased[204,205] with cheaper foods, which tend to be more energy dense and less nutritionally beneficial,[206] becoming more readily available.[207] The increasing trend in eating away from home[208–210] is expected to continue in most high-income countries.[10]

Concurrently it has been suggested that in a number of developed countries there has been a decrease in physical activity, particularly through forms such as active transport[25,211] and occupational activity[206] with the development of technology in and outside of the work place[212–214] with cars, television and computer games all affecting physical activity behaviours in recent decades.[211,215] At the same time the working population employed in the service sector, in which work is more sedentary, has increased with decreases in occupations demanding more active work such as the agricultural and the industrial sectors.[10]

In this section we discuss both micro- and macro-environmental factors which have influenced obesity.

### Microenvironmental

A microenvironment is a setting in which groups of people gather for specific purposes; these can often involve food, physical activity or both. Microenvironments are usually geographically distinct and relatively small. They can be influenced by other microenvironments as individuals can take experiences from one microenvironment into another; in doing so they transfer beliefs, attitudes and habits.

Urbanisation has been associated with more obesogenic environments through less activity promoting environments and greater access to processed foods.[4,216] Urban people live a more sedentary life, requiring less energy than those living in rural areas. Factors such as the number of recreational facilities, safety concerns in terms of crime and traffic, uneven and hilly terrain, insufficient lighting, more noise or pollution can all affect people's likelihood of being physically active in their residential environment.[217–221] Perceived risk on the roads has also been found to lead to less cycling and walking and areas designed for motorised vehicles can lead to more transport by powered rather than active transport.[10]

Urban areas also provide less healthy and more high-density foods, such as the traditional fast-food restaurants,[222] than rural areas. An increasingly high density of fast-food restaurants, convenience stores, bars, food distribution programmes with high-fat foods, and concentrated media marketing, all promote unhealthy food choices and hinder good nutrition.[223] This is not a straightforward relationship, however, as cheaper food is found in urban areas[224] with studies suggesting that people's diets are linked to the supply of food in nearby grocery stores.[225] An increased distance to supermarkets and convenience stores is associated with a poorer quality of diet[225,226] suggesting that much of the link between urbanisation and obesity may be due to area deprivation. Poorer neighbourhoods have three times fewer supermarkets than wealthier neighbourhoods, but contain more fast-food restaurants and convenience stores, limiting the availability of nearby healthy food choices.[223]

In line with the link between obesity and individual SES, poorer communities tend to be more obesogenic[227–232] and are associated with obesity independently of individual SES.[233] The deprivation of a neighbourhood is associated with characteristics of the food[234–238] and physical activity environment[234,236,239–242] which influence behaviour.[243] Such communities, where the restricted selection of food products offered limits food choices, are referred to as 'food deserts'.[244] Individuals who live in more deprived neighbourhoods feel that they are less able to use space to be active due to the lack of facilities[245] and they have worries about safety.[246,247]

Settings such as schools and workplaces are also important parts of the microenvironment which may influence dietary and activity behaviours. Variations are found in school food services[248] with school foods in some countries offering nutritionally imbalanced meals.[249,250] There has also been an increase in the availability of 'competitive food' sold through such channels as cafeterias, vending machines, a la carte meals and tuck shops or kiosks[251] which have been linked to higher consumption of unhealthy food and drinks and lower intake of healthy fresh foods.[252–254] Similarly in the workplace, vending machines stocked with energy-dense snacks are often the only option for accessing food at work[10] with the type of work affecting employees' dietary habits such as shift work, which can alter food intake patterns, resulting in less healthy diets.[255]

## Macroenvironmental

Macroenvironmental factors include the anonymous infrastructure that may influence behaviours. Indeed obesogenic environments arise through business and government reaction to economic and political environments. These include government and local policies, taxation, food production, distribution and marketing as well as the media.[151]

### Economic development

Increased wealth and increased inequality are both drivers for obesity;[5] economic growth leads to more consumption whilst technological development leads to more processed, cheaper calories.[109,256] In addition economic developments in urban areas have also led to more individuals needing to work, such that a homemaker role is less likely adopted in families, leading to decreases in time spent on preparing food and a greater demand for processes products.[10]

### Food taxes

Agriculture policies profoundly affect food consumption patterns because they give incentives for producing certain foods by providing market support[10] (Box 4.1). Trade policies are then fundamentally linked with agriculture policies, because they are

---

**Box 4.1 Case study: The EU Common Agricultural Policy**

The EU Common Agricultural Policy was created in 1962 at a time when Europe suffered from food shortages following the Second World War. The policy offered incentives to keep farmers on their land, although its original goals may not be applicable to current needs. For example, the market organisation of fruit and vegetables includes a withdrawal measure aimed at keeping prices up by limiting availability in times of seasonal overproduction, in order to protect European farmers from competition. This is compounded by widely varying import tariffs to protect the domestic market, both of which lead to an increase in price to the consumer for foods such as fruit and vegetables.[257]

Similarly the EU common market organisation for milk grants export subsidies and consumption aids to the food industry, which uses surplus butter in ice cream and pastry, decreases the cost of these products and increases their availability. Additionally without sugar subsidies, there would probably be no production of sugar in the EU and world market prices would increase by around 20%. These sugar subsidies therefore actually lead to overproduction, which in turn lowers the world market price, which eventually increases consumption worldwide. Reform agreed in the EU in February 2006 implies a 36% cut in the guaranteed minimum sugar price, compensation for farmers and a restructuring fund to encourage uncompetitive sugar producers to leave the industry such that EU production is expected to fall.[10]

---

often necessary to keep domestic agriculture support programmes in place.[10] Policies such as these may have had unintended impacts on obesity-related behaviours such as subsidies to producers which may have raised the relative prices of healthy foods, such as fruit and vegetables, and lowered the relative price of less healthy foods, such as fats and sugar.[4,258] International trade policies may have played a similar role in certain cases.[4,259]

## Urban design

Town planning, including design of the built environment and traffic regulation in many countries may have discouraged active transport in favour of motor vehicle transport[4] and lead to urbanisation linked to the spread of obesity.[4,216] Design elements in the built environment including street layout, zoning, the location of recreation and shopping facilities and services, parks and buildings and the transport system can all encourage or discourage active living.[260] From an urban and neighbourhood development perspective, the two main driving factors influencing physical activity: (i) the increasing geographical separation of living, working and shopping; and (ii) leisure activities, result in an increasing demand for motorised transport and reduce the opportunities for physically active use of the neighbourhood. Long distances to travel lead to a dependency on motorised transport with the development of towns to allow for this type of transport, making them less amenable for active transport.[220,261,262]

## Food industry

The globalisation of food has led to food becoming a commodity, meaning that products are increasingly developed on profit margins. Industrial food systems leading to mass production changed the quality and availability of food over time and affected price and convenience.[4,256] They also led to greater food storage and production, leading to diets increasingly dependent on processed and pre-packaged foods which are more energy dense and less nutritious. Decline in the price of food in the market has also led the industry to produce value-added foods, resulting in more processing, including the adding of sugar and fat.[263] Indeed some authors have suggested that the food market is failing children by making healthy choices difficult.[5] The power in the food industry has also become concentrated into an increasingly smaller number of multinational companies, which in turn increases the influence of these on government policy.[10]

The changes in food have also led to a development in the marketing of it as a produce, leading to a more focused approach in the marketing of foods.[4,264–266] There has been a development of persuasive and expensive campaigns, along with the promotion of larger portions. The position of foods within shops, special offers, branding, food packaging, marketing campaigns and many other approaches have been used to promote fatty and sugary foods which are cheaper to produce and therefore lead to high profit margins.[267] Several studies have indicated that food advertising and marketing are associated with children showing more favourable attitudes, preferences and behaviour towards the products advertised.[268,269] There are findings that even exposure to advertisements as brief as 30 seconds can significantly influence the food preferences of children as young as 2 years.[270] The range of places available for advertising has also widened with the development of technology including that found on television and in the new media, such as the internet and text messaging, on top of the development of advertising on screens in public areas and transport.[10] This has also occurred through the sponsorship of facilities such as school workbooks that contain advertising for soft drinks and snack food brands and branding in the sponsorship of sport.[271]

### Thinking points

1. Which influences can lead to an area becoming a food desert?
2. What factors can be controlled to counter the impact of urbanisation on obesity?
3. How can taxes found at a macrolevel influence what individuals choose to eat?
4. Has the globalisation of food led to any positive outcomes for the consumer?

### Summary points

- An increase in adipose tissue in the body comes as a result of an energy imbalance where energy taken in has been greater than energy used over a period of time.
- Energy intake is determined by the type and quantity of food eaten.
- A number of feedback mechanisms within the body regulate the energy taken in.
- The energy expenditure of an individual is determined by their basal metabolic rate, adaptive thermogenesis and the energy expended through physical activity.
- Although there is a genetic link to obesity, the genes interact with the environment to encourage weight gain.
- A number of early age influences have been found to influence future obesity risk.
- Individuals with lower socioeconomic status are at a greater risk of obesity.
- Individuals from minority ethnic groups are more likely to engage in obesogenic behaviours.
- Food preference can be influenced by the environment.
- Stress can have a bidirectional relationship with obesity.
- Parents, peers and spouses are all linked to BMI.
- Social convention and religious practices both influence obesogenic behaviours.
- Urbanisation has been associated with more obesogenic environments.
- Resource-poorer communities tend to be more obesogenic and associated with obesity independently of individual socioeconomic status.
- Policies created to protect business can encourage less healthy behaviours.
- The globalisation of food has led to food becoming a commodity, meaning that products are increasingly developed on profit margins.

## Web pages and resources

National Obesity Observatory 'Causes of Obesity' with Foresight full obesity system map.
www.noo.org.uk/NOO_about_obesity/causes.
Foresight. Tackling Obesities: future Choices – Project Report. 2nd ed.
www.bis.gov.uk/assets/foresight/docs/obesity/17.pdf.
Rand Health Research on Food Environments and Obesity.
www.rand.org/health/feature/food-environment-obesity.html.

CDC. Obesity & Genetics,
www.cdc.gov/features/obesity.

## Further reading

1. Cutler, et al. Why have Americans Become More Obese? National Bureau of Economic Research; 2003.
   *This paper describes trends in obesity in the United States along with changes in energy consumed and expended, going on to discuss the role of technological and economic development on obesity*

*in the US. They also consider changes across population subgroups and other countries.*

2. Rolls. Understanding the mechanisms of food intake and obesity. Obes Rev 2007;8(Suppl. 1): 67–72.
*This review considers the brain mechanisms which control appetite along with a number of sensory and environmental factors which can override these feedback mechanisms and lead to over consumption.*

3. Swinburn, et al. The global obesity pandemic: shaped by global drivers and local environments. Lancet 2011;378:804–14.
*This paper describes the obesity epidemic and explains the reasons for its concurrent rise across countries, as well as the wide variation in obesity prevalence between countries.*

# 5 Individual interventions to treat obesity

Any intervention that is to encourage weight loss should lead to greater energy expenditure than energy intake and any long-term treatment must involve some form of lifestyle change.[1] As the causes of obesity are so numerous and diverse, there is unlikely to be a 'one-size-fits-all' intervention to target obesity on an individual level.[2,3] The right intervention for an individual will be determined by a number of factors including sex, age and ethnicity.[3] There are a range of guidelines produced which help health professionals deal with overweight patients and recommend a course of treatment or intervention, such as: Scottish Intercollegiate Guidelines Network,[4] the United States National Institutes of Health,[5] the Royal College of Physicians of London,[6] the National Health and Medical Research Council of Australia[2] and the National Institute for Health and Clinical Excellence.[7]

## Consultation

Individuals may not initially present about weight loss, so the health professional may need to raise the subject;[2] conversely not every individual who seeks weight loss advice actually needs it.[8] Screening and assessment are therefore important in initial consultations. NICE recommend that after the appropriate measurements are taken to assess obesity risk (see Chapter 1) a follow-up assessment should be conducted covering the following areas:[7]

- Presenting symptoms and underlying causes of excess weight.
- Lifestyle assessment including dietary and activity behaviour.
- Unhelpful beliefs towards obesity re-lated behaviours, including culturally specific beliefs.
- Previous experience in weight loss and outcomes.
- Any comorbidities or risk factors the individual exhibits including:

type 2 diabetes, hypertension, cardiovascular disease, osteoarthritis, dyslipidaemia and sleep apnoea.

- Psychosocial distress along with lifestyle, environmental, social and family factors which may lead to obesity, such as a family history of overweight and obesity and/or comorbidities.
- An assessment of a willingness and motivation to change lifestyle to lose weight, along with confidence that changes can be made.
- The potential of any weight loss to improve the health of the individual.
- Any psychological problems the individual displays.
- Any medical problems the individual suffers or medication they are taking.

Similar assessments should be conducted with children, for whom growth and pubertal status should also be considered, and the issue of weight raised with both the child and their family.[7]

This screening of obesity and associated risk factors, along with risk factors for CVD can help to target an intervention for the individual.[9–11] These can be either brief interventions which require little time,[12–14] or referral to more specialist care. Even where initial consultation results in referral to more specialised interventions, this initial interaction can help motivate the patient throughout the treatment.[15]

Brief interventions should be planned and consistent and include the following stages:[16,17] (1) screening; (2) counselling; (3) referral; and (4) follow-up.

## 1. Screening to identify risk and willingness to change

Initial screening should be individual even if follow-up interventions are in groups.[18] Health professionals should follow the usual principles of person-centred care, with the individual provided an opportunity to make informed decisions about their treatment, in partnership with their health professionals.[7] Staff should avoid assumptions and should allow modification of treatment based on feedback. Advice, treatment and care should take into account people's needs and preferences, adapting the approach to encourage participation, self-esteem and self-efficacy.[5,19] This is particularly important for MEGs, vulnerable groups (such as those on low incomes) and people at life stages with increased risk for weight gain. Advice should be non-discriminatory, culturally appropriate and accessible to people with additional needs, such as physical, sensory or learning disabilities.[7]

The possible aims for treatments of overweight and obesity should be negotiated and documented with each individual. These could include:[8]

1. Realistic weight loss.
2. A decrease in waist circumference.
3. Changes in body composition.
4. Alleviation of related metabolic disease.
5. Alleviation of related mechanical disease.
6. Increased activity.
7. Decreased use of medications.

8. Improved quality of life, well-being and psychosocial functioning.
9. Improved fertility if relevant.
10. Other individual goals which can include weight loss for a special occasion.

Not all individuals are ready for change and for those who appear resistant it can be helpful to assist them to explore their ambivalence in a non-judgmental way,[20] whilst barriers to lifestyle change are explored. These may include:[7]

- Lack of knowledge or skill.
- Financial costs of behaviour change.
- Safety concerns.
- Time constraints.
- Personal preference.
- Social influence.
- Low baseline fitness, or disabilities.
- Low self-esteem or assertiveness.

Individuals who are not ready to change should be offered the chance to return for further consultations and given information on the benefits of losing weight, healthy eating and increased physical activity.[7]

In secondary care, the assessment of overweight and/or obese children and young people should also include assessment of associated comorbidities and possible aetiology. These should include measurements for blood pressure, fasting lipid profile, fasting insulin and glucose levels, liver and endocrine function. Results should be interpreted in the context of the degree of overweight and obesity, the child's age, history of comorbidities, possible genetic causes and any family history of metabolic disease related to overweight and obesity.[7]

### 2. Counselling to provide information and increase motivation

Individuals who are overweight or obese, and their families and/or carers, should be given relevant information on:[7]

- Overweight and obesity in general, including related health risks.
- Realistic short- and long-term targets for weight loss.
- The distinction between losing weight and maintaining weight loss.
- Realistic targets other than weight loss, such as behaviour change.
- Diagnosis and treatment options.
- Healthy eating in general.
- Medication and side effects.
- Surgical treatments and drug therapy.
- Self-care.
- Voluntary organisations and support groups and how to contact them.

Although individual counselling for weight management can be delivered by a range of health professionals[18] this should be done by those with the relevant competence and experience. Training of health professionals should include:[7]

1. Health benefits and potential effectiveness of interventions to prevent obesity and promote behaviour change.
2. Best practice in delivering interventions, including tailoring support to individual's needs in the long term.
3. The use of motivational interviewing (MI) and counselling techniques.

For professionals with little or no experience of MI or individual counselling, it may be necessary to offer more generic communication skills training before focusing on counselling skills.[20]

### 3. Referral for those at high risk to intervention

As obesity is a complex condition it requires a multidisciplinary input. Clinicians should work with specialist health professionals such as dieticians, exercise physiologists or specialist obesity physicians[21] to encourage weight loss.[9–11] Referral to specialist care should be considered for any of the following:[7]

- The underlying causes of overweight and obesity are not clear and need further assessment.
- Individual has complex disease states and/or needs that cannot be managed adequately in primary or secondary care.
- Conventional treatment has failed.
- Specialist interventions may be required.
- Drug therapy or surgical intervention is being considered.

Referral to an appropriate specialist should also be considered for children who are overweight or obese and have significant comorbidity, or complex needs such as educational difficulties.[7]

### 4. Follow-up to track progress and overcome barriers

Weight gain often follows weight loss so individuals attempting weight loss should have long-term contact and support from health professionals.[22] Weight loss should be approached incrementally with new goals set when the original target has been reached.[8] Long-term follow-up is very important for successful outcomes[23,24] with frequent contact between health professionals and individuals found to promote weight loss and maintenance, with the amount of time spent with a patient enhancing this.[5] Arrangements should also be made for transitional care for young people who are moving from paediatric to adult services.[7]

> **! Thinking points**
>
> 1. What are the challenges of a multidisciplinary approach?
> 2. What approach should be taken with individuals wishing to lose weight who do not need to?
> 3. What factors indicate the need for referral to specialist care?
> 4. What approach should be taken for individuals who don't want to lose weight?

## Adult interventions

Although well-designed interventions can be applicable to many people, any approach should be targeted to the individual.[17] However, all interventions should be multicomponent, focusing on diet and physical activity together, and include a behavioural component[25–28] as these are more effective than interventions which focus on one behaviour,[2,7,20] particularly in the long term.[5,29]

Initial weight loss or behavioural goals should be achievable and short-term,[18,30] set with the individual[7] and consider initial BMI.[20] Advice suggests that a weight loss of around 0.5 to 1.0 kg each week[5,7] with an initial maximum target of 10% of body weight was found to be suitable, as this has significant impacts on health risks.[8] Unrealistic expectations of weight loss by the individual should be moderated[2] as obese patients often expect to lose a great deal more than is realistic and recommended.[31,32]

Initial weight loss can often plateau or reverse due to physiological adaptation[33] so a maintenance programme is important.[5] For behaviour change to be sustained, several follow-up sessions after the initial consultation are important with more frequent and/or longer contact sessions associated with greater reductions in body mass and improvements in physical activity and diet.[34–36] The level of support should be adaptable and determined by the individual's needs[7] with self-monitoring and self-regulation found to be important.[18,37]

## Non-clinical interventions targeting obesity

Although there is little evidence of interventions in non-clinical settings to produce sustainable weight loss, there is some suggestion that multicomponent commercial weight loss programmes may be more effective than self-help programmes[38] with support thought to be an important factor.[20] NICE recommends that primary care organisations and local authorities should only recommend self-help, commercial and community weight management programmes if they follow best practice by:[7]

- Helping assess weight and determine realistic targets.
- Aim for a reasonable and safe weekly weight loss.
- Focus on long-term lifestyle changes, not short-term weight loss.
- Are multicomponent, addressing both diet and activity.
- Follow a balanced, healthy-eating approach.
- Encourage regular physical activity as a part of daily life along with practical, safe advice.
- Include behaviour change techniques, such as self-monitoring and coping with lapses.
- Recommend or provide on-going support.

The WHO provide a table of measures which can be used to judge the success of anti-obesity treatments (Table 5.1).

## Diet

Dietary interventions should aim to improve diet and reduce energy intake, bringing together a number of components such as dietary modification, targeted advice, family involvement and goal setting. These should be individualised, tailored to food preferences and allow for

**Table 5.1** Process measures to judge the success of anti-obesity treatment

| MEASURES | BENEFITS | |
| --- | --- | --- |
| | Immediate | Longer-term |
| **Physical** | Weight loss | Reduced breathlessness |
| | Reduction in waist circumference | Decreased sleep apnoea |
| **Metabolic** | Improvements in co-morbidities | Reduced angina |
| | Decreased fasting blood glucose and plasma insulin | Reduced blood pressure |
| | Improvement in fasting lipid profile | Reduction in doses on concomitant medications |
| | Decreased glycosylated haemoglobin level if diabetic | |
| **Functional** | Increased mobility | Reduced time away from work |
| | Decreased symptoms | Improved involvement in social activities |
| | Increased well-being and mood | Fewer consultations with health professionals |
| | Increased health-related quality of life | |

*Source: WHO [2007] The Challenge of obesity in the WHO European Region and the strategies for response.*

flexible approaches to reducing calorie intake, and for overall success must be sustainable for the long term.[39,40] This should lead to a diet that follows healthy eating advice, as low-calorie diets are less likely to be nutritionally complete.[20] NICE recommends a few dietary changes which should be incorporated into a diet to encourage weight loss with:[7]

- Meals based on starchy and fibre-rich foods, including wholegrain where possible.
- At least five portions of a variety of fruit and vegetables every day, in place of foods higher in fat and calories rather than as well as.
- Reductions in the amount of fat and added sugar. In particular as little as possible of fried foods, sugary drinks and confectionery.
- Daily breakfast.
- Portion control for meals and snacks.
- Minimal energy taken in the form of alcohol.

Diets should only be followed when combined with expert support and intensive follow-up[5] or clinical supervision where major reductions in energy intake have been made.[20]

Although these is some evidence of the success for popular diets such as the Mediterranean[41,42] or

GI diet[43] these findings are not consistent[44,45] with some, such as the low-carbohydrate high-protein diets, suggested to increase CVD risk.[46]

The main types of diet commonly recommended to encourage weight loss include reduced-energy diets, low-energy diets, very-low-energy diets and fixed-energy-deficit diets.[2,7]

**Reduced-energy diet (RED)** REDs do not set a specific energy level but reduce current intake, often through reducing fat intake, which can encourage weight loss and lead to improvements in CVD risk.[47] REDs have been found to lead to loss of body weight of around 4% over one to two years[2,48,49] with decreases in levels of abdominal fat and in waist circumference.[2] As compliance is improved in comparison to more prescriptive diets, they may prove more effective at maintaining weight loss.[50] The amount of energy reduction required to achieve weight loss varies by a number of individual factors including age, sex and current behaviour.

**Low-energy diet (LED)** LEDs reduce an individual's energy intake to around 1200 kilocalories or lower a day. These lead to quicker weight loss than REDs, but are only suitable for higher-risk individuals.[50] LEDs should not be considered for continuous long-term treatment and should only be undertaken with close expert supervision.[2,7] As these diets are very prescriptive, they are unlikely to be sustained for the long term and must be combined with other lifestyle changes to maintain weight loss.

**Very-low-energy diets (VLED)** VLEDs involve daily energy intake of around 800 kilocalories a day and lower. They can lead to quick, short-term weight loss, but individuals must be closely monitored throughout. They can only be used in the short term (eight to 16 weeks) and only for those with life-threatening comorbidities. They must contain 0.8 to 1.0 grams of protein per kilogram of ideal body weight and provide recommended amounts of minerals, vitamins, trace elements and essential fatty acids. VLEDs should not be used for extended periods, with evidence suggesting they do not provide better long-term outcomes than less rigid diets. After finishing the diet, food should be carefully reintroduced.[2,7]

**Fixed-energy-deficit (FED)** FEDs provide a structured eating plan, based on an individual's energy requirements, estimated by calculating BMR and adjusting for levels of activity. An energy deficit of around 600 kcal a day is developed to induce weight loss of around 0.5 kg per week. FEDs are less prescriptive and extreme than both LEDs and VLEDs which may improve compliance and are recommended for sustainable weight loss.[7]

## Physical activity

Although there is a linear dose relationship between physical activity and weight loss[51,52] physical activity interventions on their own do not seem to encourage as much weight loss as dietary interventions, unless the physical activity is at very high levels.[53] Increases in activity, however, have been found to encourage decreases in abdominal fat and play a role in long-term weight maintenance, as well as improving cardiorespiratory fitness. Individuals are therefore encouraged to increase their physical activity level even in the absence of significant losses in body weight[2] with some suggesting that it is more important to prevent inactivity or sedentary behaviour.[54] It must also be remembered that physical activity can preserve or increase fat-free mass, which must be accounted for when weight loss is an aim of any intervention.[55,56]

Evidence suggests that the form of physical activity that most effectively improves metabolic health is moderate-intensity aerobic activity carried out regularly over an extended period.[2] Recommended levels of physical activity vary, but generally involve 30 minutes of moderate activity on at least 5 days of the week, although it is thought that periods longer than 30 minutes are generally required in order to prevent weight regain, with more vigorous exercise also recommended.[57] Resistance training activities are also thought to be beneficial, particularly in older individuals who may suffer muscle wastage.[58,59]

The physical activity component of interventions should be tailored to the individual and focus on activities that fit easily into their lives if they are to sustain and encourage long-term weight loss.[2] Prior to intervention a fitness assessment should be performed to ensure the individual is safe to increase activity levels.[2] For very large patients, with some degree of immobility, a reduced weight-bearing form of activity may be best in the early stages of an intervention, until their fitness increases and weight-bearing activities can be more easily carried out.[2]

## Behavioural

Weight management and weight loss are improved by implementing strategies that provide tools for overcoming barriers to compliance with diet therapy or increased physical activity.[43] For optimal results, aspects of behavioural therapy should be combined with nutrition and exercise therapy[2] as the most effective lifestyle approach to managing weight[26,28] by sustaining behaviour change in the long term.[25,27] However, a cessation of behavioural therapy can lead to weight gain,[5] often to the initial weight.[60,61] Maintenance of weight loss requires continuous care[25] with behavioural treatment combined with post-treatment contact with a therapist leading to greater long-term weight loss.[62]

Behavioural strategies can include psychological aspects of motivation, stress management, relapse prevention, counselling, and techniques such as hypnosis and psychotherapy.[2] Behavioural therapy should also be considered for psychological conditions associated with obesity-related behaviours such as depression[63] or stress.[64–66] A behavioural intervention which has attracted a lot of attention is motivational interviewing (MI). MI is a collaborative, person-centred form of guiding to elicit and strengthen motivation for change[67] often delivered over an extended time period.[68] The principles of MI are illustrated by the acronym RULE:[69]

**R:** Resist the righting reflex. Avoid the inclination to correct the individual's behaviour.

**U:** Understand and explore the individual's motivations.

**L:** Listen with empathy.

**E:** Empower the individual, encourage hope and optimism.

MI has been found to have some effect[34] through enhancing weight loss.[70] It takes longer than giving direct advice[43,71] and should only be delivered by those with the appropriate training, which follows a sequence of eight stages and requires a minimum of two days, followed by on-going supervision and follow-up training.[72,73]

The evidence on which behavioural therapy works best is limited and any approach should be chosen through the requirements of the individual as part of a multimodal strategy.[5] It has been recommended that behavioural interventions for adults should include the following strategies, as appropriate for the person:[2,5,7]

- Self-monitoring of body weight and behaviour.[74,75]
- Goal setting.
- Decreased eating rate.
- Stress management, coping and relaxation strategies.
- Assertiveness training.
- Stimulus control.[76]
- Problem solving in reflection of failure.[77]
- Contingency management through self-rewards for achieving goals.
- Reinforcement of changes.
- Cognitive restructuring to modify inaccurate beliefs that undermine weight loss efforts.[78,79]
- Relapse prevention.
- Strategies for dealing with weight gain.
- Social support.[80,81]

> **! Thinking points**
>
> 1. Why is it important to moderate unrealistic expectations of weight loss?
> 2. What are the risks associated with low- and very-low-energy diets?
> 3. How can measurements be taken which account for changes in muscle when undergoing a physical activity intervention?
> 4. What benefits does behavioural therapy bring to a multicomponent intervention?

## Child interventions

Weight management should start in childhood for overweight and obese individuals. Interventions with children should also be multicomponent and targeted to the individual, considering factors such as age and maturity. Interventions should include dietary modification, increased physical activity, decreased sedentary activity, family involvement, and behaviour modification.[21]

Targets for children differ from adults, because absolute weight loss is not always necessary in young children as some may grow into their weight if it is maintained. Changes can then be judged against BMI from growth charts, with the weight percentile moving closer to the height percentile.[21] Other outcomes may focus on behaviours[82] or the alleviation of obesity-related illness.[8] At the same time the stigmatisation of treating obese children should be considered, such that confidentiality and building self-esteem and body image are particularly important.[7]

Weight loss in adolescence can differ from that in childhood as this is a time which involves a number of conflicting issues to conventional management interventions, such as independence from family and conformity with one's peer group.[83] Adolescents are less likely to accept a highly prescriptive intervention and are more likely to resist treatment. This can mean that adolescents fall in between paediatric and adult services, as they refuse to be treated as children but are less reliable than adults.[8] Additionally, whereas in children weight maintenance may be the primary goal, older adolescents have lost height growth as a means of

weight reduction, and puberty may have already exacerbated the degree of overweight.[83]

For both children and adolescents, there is evidence that weight-management programmes that involve parents achieve better outcomes. This can include overcoming parental barriers such as a refusal to acknowledge that their child requires treatment.[8] For children of primary school age, there is also evidence that a programme that involves parents alone does better than one that also requires regular attendance by their children. Parents can alter environments substantially, especially for younger children,[21] and parenting skills are an important part of any intervention in child obesity.[84] Some also suggest that parent-focused interventions help children overcome resistance to change and distract from the stigmatisation of being identified as obese.[85] The involvement of parents can differ by age of child, although the social setting should be considered for all children.[7,8] With younger children, family group treatment is more important than for adolescents, for whom individual treatment may be more appropriate,[7,8] with a balance found between the importance of involving parents and the right of the child to be cared for independently.[7]

Dietary control in children can have negative consequences, including loss of lean body mass, reduced height growth and an exacerbation of eating disorders, so weight-maintenance is preferred for all but very obese children until after puberty. For very obese children or moderately obese children with additional health complications, a balanced low-energy diet that uses normally available foods is recommended.[8] Children and young adults should eat regular meals, including breakfast, in a pleasant, sociable environment without distractions, and parents and carers should eat with children, with all family members eating the same foods.[7]

Active play should be encouraged[7] with activity integrated into the life of the individual.[8] Families should try to be more active as a unit. Sedentary behaviour should be reduced gradually and replaced with active alternatives, which may be outside of the home, such as at school or clubs.[7]

Behavioural interventions which can also be used with children include:

- Stimulus control.
- Self-monitoring.
- Goal setting.
- Rewards for reaching goals.
- Problem solving.[7]
- Cognitive behavioural therapy.
- Family therapy.[8]

Drugs and surgical interventions are not recommended for children[8] and referral to an appropriate specialist should be considered for children who have significant comorbidity or complex needs, such as learning difficulties.[7] This can include referral to specialised schools or hospital treatment.[8]

> ### ! Thinking points
>
> 1. What factors must be considered when deciding whether weight loss or weight maintenance should be the primary goal of the intervention?
> 2. How should interventions differ when treating children and adolescents?
> 3. What approaches can be taken when parents do not agree that their child needs to lose weight?
> 4. Why is it important to consider the pubertal status of the individual in any assessment?

## Drug therapy

Many obese individuals increasingly believe that drugs and surgery are the only effective treatment options.[5] This idea that medical intervention is required to enable weight loss disempowers the individual and diminishes a sense of self-efficacy in weight maintenance. At the same time if these interventions became the standard treatment of obesity it would result in a huge impact on the health economies of many countries and may prove unsustainable. Robust criteria must therefore be used to assess which individuals are suitable for drug or surgical intervention[8] and both should only be considered for the very obese or for those who suffer the medical complications of obesity.

## Anti-obesity drugs

Pharmacological treatment should only be considered for individuals with impaired health, who have been unsuccessful in losing weight by other means. With criteria set for the selection of suitable individuals:[5,86,87]

1. A BMI greater than 30 kg/m$^2$ if they display no concomitant obesity-related risk factors or diseases, or greater than 27 kg/m$^2$ with concomitant obesity-related risk factors or diseases; and
2. History of a failure to lose weight on a programme of diet, exercise and behavioural therapy.

Drugs should not be used in isolation and should only be considered in conjunction with interventions that target behaviour change.[88] The decision to start any drug therapy should only be made after a full discussion with the individual around the potential benefits and limitations of the treatment. Assessment of suitable individuals should also consider the potentials for drug abuse, meaning that continuing regulation is important with information, support and counselling provided throughout the course of treatment.[7] If the drug proves effective in aiding or sustaining weight loss and there are no serious adverse effects, it can be continued; if not, it should be discontinued.[5]

The two general classes of anti-obesity drugs currently in use include those that work within the bowel to restrict fat absorption and centrally acting drugs that suppress appetite.[3] In order for any drug to be permitted for use they must be approved by the regulatory authority of that country. Information on the drugs currently approved for use, or on the current position of specific drugs, along with guidance on prescribing and treatment, can be found through websites of the regulatory organisations (Box 5.1). Organisations such as NIH, NHMRC or NICE will also provide guidance on their use.

It is important that current advice on recommended treatments is regularly followed, as past recommendations have been withdrawn in light of new evidence (see Box 5.2). Individuals should also be advised on the lack of evidence for the use of alternative, over-the-counter weight-loss medications

---

**Box 5.1 Drug and treatment regulatory authorities**

**Australia** – Therapeutic Goods Administration:
www.tga.gov.au/
**Canada** – Therapeutic Products Directorate (TPD) of Health Canada:
www.hc-sc.gc.ca
**Europe** – European Medicines Agency:
www.ema.europa.eu/ema/
**New Zealand** – New Zealand Medicines and Medical Devices Safety Authority:
www.medsafe.govt.nz/
**USA** – US Food and Drug Administration:
www.fda.gov/
**UK** – Medicines and Healthcare products Regulatory Authority:
www.mhra.gov.uk

---

**Box 5.2 Case study: Sibutramine approval withdrawn**

Sibutramine, traded under a number of names (Ectiva/Meridia/Raductil/Reductil/Sibutral Reductil®), was a serotonin and noradrenaline re-uptake inhibitor which was thought to promote a sense of satiety[8,21] and had been found to encourage weight loss, decrease visceral fat and improve obesity-related risk factors.[89–96]

Sibutramine was FDA-approved in 1997 for weight loss and weight maintenance.[97] It was also approved for use in many countries including the UK and Australia.[98] However, in 2010 new data from the Sibutramine Cardiovascular Outcomes Trial (SCOUT)[99,100] demonstrated an increase in risk of major adverse cardiovascular events in individuals treated with it. In reaction the FDA, MHRA in Europe[101] and the TGA in Australia[102] concluded that the risks from the drug outweighed any benefit from the modest weight loss and withdrew approval for it use.[97]

These organisations now recommend:

- No new prescriptions for sibutramine should be issued and the current use of the drug with every individual should be reviewed.
- Pharmacists should not dispense the drug and advise those individuals hoping to receive it to make an appointment to see their clinician.
- Individuals currently using the drug should make a routine appointment with their clinician to discuss alternative measures to lose weight, including use of diet and exercise regimens. Individuals may stop treatment before their appointment if they wish.

---

and, in some cases, the possible dangers of their use.[2] Additionally, although there has been use of drug therapy with adolescents in specialist centres, in general the use of drugs with children or adolescents is not recommended.[21]

## Lipase inhibitors

The most commonly used inhibitor is Orlistat (Xenical®), the only drug in this class with efficacy and safety supported by clinical evidence.[2] It is approved for use in most countries.[103] Orlistat acts by inhibiting pancreatic and gastric lipase, leading to decreased hydrolysis of ingested triglycerides.[8] It is not absorbed and acts entirely in the lumen of the small intestine where it is thought to reduce fat absorption by around 30%.[103]

Orlistat has been found to lead to weight loss and improvements in CVD risk factors when used in conjunction with behaviour change interventions.[48,104–111] As Orlistat inhibits fat absorption this can lead to steatorrhoea and diarrhoea if individuals eat fatty foods, with individuals advised to keep their fat intake below 20 grams per meal, to minimise adverse gastrointestinal effects.[86] It therefore not only contributes to weight loss by reducing fat absorption, but also leads to behaviour change by encouraging individuals to avoid fat in their diet.

However, it has been recommended that individuals on Orlistat require regular monitoring amidst concerns that many patients are left on the drug even when there is no evidence of weight loss.[112]

## Appetite suppressants

In 2012 the US Food and Drug Administration (FDA) approved the use of two appetite suppressants Qsymia® and Belviq®, the first anti-obesity drugs to be approved for over a decade. Both drugs have been found to encourage weight loss as part of a multicomponent intervention and are approved for use as an addition to a reduced-calorie diet and exercise regimen for chronic weight management in adults who fulfil the criteria described above. Although they are not approved for use in the UK, Australasia or Canada their use is currently under review in Europe.[113,114]

Qsymia is a combination of two FDA-approved drugs, phentermine, an appetite suppressant, and topiramate, which is indicated to treat certain types of seizures in epileptics and to prevent migraine headaches. Together they are thought to target brain mechanisms which trigger overeating.[115]

The FDA warn that Qsymia must not be used during pregnancy, due to the risk of foetal defects such as oral clefts. Women of reproductive potential should have a negative pregnancy test before starting therapy and every month during it. Additionally Qsymia must not be used in patients with glaucoma or hyperthyroidism. The use of Qsymia in patients with recent or unstable heart disease or stroke is not recommended, as it increases heart rate, whilst regular monitoring of heart rate is recommended for all patients especially when starting therapy or increasing dose.[115]

Belviq (lorcaserin hydrochloride) works by activating serotonin 2C receptors in the brain which may promote feelings of satiety. A side effect of Belviq could include serotonin syndrome, particularly when taken with certain medicines which increase serotonin levels or activate serotonin receptors, such as anti-depressants or migraine treatments. Because preliminary data suggest that the number of serotonin 2B receptors may be increased in patients with congestive heart failure, Belviq should be used with caution in patients with this condition. As with Qsymi, Belviq should not be used during pregnancy.[116]

## Surgical intervention

There are a number of surgical interventions used to reduce stomach volume, referred to as bariatric surgery. They are commonly performed laparoscopically (using keyhole techniques) although they can also be done through open surgery. No differences have been found between these two approaches in weight outcomes, but open surgery is more risky[117] and more likely to lead to infections and other conditions. Laparoscopic methods also mean a reduction in the length of recovery and post-operative stays in hospital, use of less analgesia and less severe physical discomfort.[118] However, re-operation can be more common[117] and can occur due to adverse events such as anastomosis leakage, pneumonia, pulmonary embolism, band slippage and band erosion. A mortality rate of 0.25% has been reported for bariatric surgery,[119] although this differs between procedures, with laparoscopic adjustable gastric banding (LAGB) found to have a lower risk than gastric by-pass (GBP).[120]

Bariatric surgery has been found to be more effective for achieving and sustaining weight loss than non-surgical management in people with severe obesity.[121–123] It has also been found to lead to marked reductions in some obesity-related co-morbidities[124] such as diabetes and hypertension which may be due to the neuroendocrine effects of surgery in addition to its restriction of food intake and/or malabsorption.[125]

However, surgery should not be viewed as an easy option, as it makes a dramatic impact on lifestyle and individuals will still have to monitor their dietary choice and activity behaviour. Malabsorption can also lead to micronutrient deficiencies, common to nearly all bariatric surgery, especially of micronutrients involved in red blood cell production and bone metabolism, necessitating supplementation and monitoring.[2] Additionally surgery is more costly than non-surgical interventions, although they may prove cost effective in those with higher BMI[126] especially for less risky procedures.[127] NICE has published a costing tool to allow an economic evaluation of offering bariatric surgery.[7]

The careful selection of individuals for surgical intervention is critical and it is not considered suitable for everyone.[128] It is recommended that surgery should only be considered under the following criteria:[5,7,129]

- A BMI greater than $40 \, \text{kg/m}^2$ if they display no concomitant obesity-related risk factors or diseases, or greater than $35 \, \text{kg/m}^2$ with concomitant obesity-related risk factors or diseases.
- It can be a first-line option for adults with a BMI $\geq 50 \, \text{kg/m}^2$ as part of a comprehensive package of obesity services provided by a multidisciplinary team.
- All appropriate non-surgical measures have been tried but have failed to achieve or maintain adequate, clinically beneficial weight loss for at least 6 months. Severely obese patients seeking therapy for the first time should initially be considered for treatment in non-surgical multicomponent programmes.

- The individual has been receiving or will receive intensive management in a specialist obesity service.
- The individual is well-informed and motivated with acceptable operative risk and selected after careful evaluation by a multidisciplinary team with medical, surgical, psychiatric, and nutritional expertise.
- The individual is generally fit for anaesthesia and surgery.
- The individual commits to the need for long-term follow-up.

The use of surgery for children and adolescents is not recommended[8] and can only ever be considered under exceptional circumstances, as the last possible option in a severely obese adolescent with obesity-related co-morbidity[2] when the individual has achieved physiological maturity.[7] Such a procedure should be undertaken only in an experienced surgical centre after extensive consultation, lengthy education of the patient and their family, and full psychological assessment with continuing post-operative care in an experienced weight-management service is mandatory. Women should also be advised to avoid pregnancy after surgery until their weight has stabilised and any micronutrient deficiencies have been identified and treated.[2]

After an individual has been referred for surgery, the choice of surgical intervention should be made jointly by the person and the clinician, taking into account the degree of obesity, any comorbidities, best available evidence on effectiveness and long-term effects, the facilities and equipment available, along with the experience of the surgeon who would perform the operation.[7] The most common forms of bariatric surgery include:[122,123,130]

1. **Laparoscopic adjustable gastric banding (LAGB or AGB):** A relatively non-invasive surgery that is easy to reverse. An adjustable band is applied to the upper stomach and creates a small pouch above the band with a narrowing between the pouch and the rest of the stomach. This reduces feelings of hunger and restricts the amount of food that can be eaten. Adjustments can be made by changing the diameter of the outlet through changing the levels of saline in a portal under the skin that is connected to the band.

2. **Laparoscopic or open Roux-en-Y gastric bypass (GBP):** Creates a small pouch from the original stomach which is connected to the oesophagus and small intestine, thereby bypassing the stomach and the initial loop of the small intestine. This affects absorption so patients may be at risk of nutritional deficiencies and therefore need lifelong supplements and monitoring. The NHMRC recommend that due to malabsorption complications, this

procedure should only be used for heavier patients.[131]

3. **Laparoscopic or open sleeve gastrectomy (SG):** Divides the stomach vertically, reducing it in size by about three quarters, thereby affecting appetite and satiety. This is not reversible and can be used as a first stage for progression to GBP or other procedures in very obese patients, where initial procedure would be technically difficult or unsafe.

4. **Laparoscopic or open biliopancreatic diversion (BPD) and duodenal switch:** All involve removal of portions of the stomach to decrease size. These are more risky than other forms of bariatric surgery, with higher mortality risk and they can result in nutritional deficiency, biochemical disruption and unpleasant side effects.

5. **The silicon intragastric balloon (IGB):** Placing an IGB in the stomach reduces volume and leads to premature feelings of satiety. This is done through an interventionist endoscopic procedure and can be used where surgery is particularly high risk, or as an interim measure.

6. **Vertical banded gastroplasty (VBG):** Gastroplasty limits the size of the stomach by stapling, or through the attachment of an external ring or adjustable band;[2]

it is now performed infrequently as it has been replaced by LAGB because of its long-term improved performance.[20]

After surgery regular, specialist postoperative dietetic monitoring should be provided. This should include information on the appropriate diet for the procedure, monitoring of the individual's micronutrient status, information on support groups, individualised nutritional supplementation, and support and guidance to achieve long-term weight loss and weight maintenance.[7]

The NIH recommend that any operation should be performed by a surgeon who has substantial experience with the procedure and is working in a clinical setting with adequate support for all aspects of management and assessment, with lifelong medical surveillance essential after surgical therapy.[129] NICE also provide recommendations for the surgery itself, recommending that it should only be undertaken by a multidisciplinary team that can provide a range services:[7]

- Preoperative assessment, including a risk–benefit analysis that includes preventing complications of obesity, and specialist assessment for eating disorder(s).
- Information on the different procedures, including potential weight loss and associated risks.

- Regular postoperative assessment, including specialist dietetic and surgical follow-up.
- Management of comorbidities.
- Psychological support before and after surgery.
- Information on, or access to, plastic surgery (such as apronectomy) where appropriate.
- Access to suitable equipment, including scales, theatre tables, Zimmer frames, commodes, hoists, bed frames, pressure-relieving mattresses and seating suitable for patients undergoing bariatric surgery, and staff trained to use them.

> **! Thinking points**
>
> 1. Why should individuals be discouraged from viewing drug or surgical interventions as a 'cure' for obesity?
> 2. Why is on-going monitoring and research into the use of weight-loss drugs important?
> 3. Why can both drug therapy and surgery be viewed as psychological as well as physiological interventions?
> 4. What factors must be considered in judging whether the benefits of surgery outweigh the risks or costs?

> **Summary points**
>
> - As obesity is a complex condition it requires a multidisciplinary input and range of interventions.
> - Individuals may not present initially about weight, but with some other condition.
> - A number of guidelines are produced informing health professionals how to deal with overweight patients.
> - Initial consultation and assessment are important in choosing the intervention approach and can influence later success.
> - Any intervention should be targeted at the individual.
> - Interventions should have dietary, activity and behavioural components.
> - Weight-loss diets should only be followed with expert support and follow-up, or clinical supervision.
> - Activities should be encouraged that easily fit into the individual's life.
> - Strict criteria should be used in the selection of individuals suitable for drug therapy or surgical intervention.
> - Both should be used with careful monitoring and alongside behaviour change interventions.
> - Neither is recommended for use with children and young people.
> - Although bariatric surgery has become safer due to the development of keyhole techniques it still carries a significant risk.

## Web pages and resources

NICE guidance on treating obesity.
http://publications.nice.org.uk/obesity-cg43.
Australian Government, National Health and
    Medical Research Council, guidelines.
http://www.nhmrc.gov.au/guidelines/
    publications/n57.
National Institutes of Health, publications on
    clinical treatment of obesity.
http://www.nhlbi.nih.gov/guidelines/obesity/
    ob_gdlns.htm.
Centers for Disease Control and Prevention,
    resources on obesity.
www.cdc.gov/obesity/resources/.

## Further reading

1. Smith, et al. Surgical approaches to the
   treatment of obesity: bariatric surgery. Medical
   Clinics of North America 2011;95:1009–30.

*Describes current types of bariatric surgery, their
outcomes and impact on obesity-related medical
comorbidities.*

2. NOO. Brief Interventions for Weight
   Management. Oxford: National Obesity
   Observatory; 2011.
   *Provides a short guide to brief interventions for
   weight management with adults.*

3. Livingston, Zylke. Progress in obesity
   research: reasons for optimism. JAMA
   2012;308(11):1162–4.
   *Summarises recent evidence on the effectiveness of
   different methods to treat obesity and encourage
   weight loss.*

---

* To view the full reference list for the book, click here http://dx.doi.org/10.1016/
B978-0-7020-4634-6.09992-1

# 6 Population approaches to preventing obesity

The individual-level interventions discussed in Chapter 5 may have some impact on individual BMI and health. However, if obesity is to be combated on a national level, much broader approaches that target whole population groups and the obesogenic environmental influences need to be in place. The aim should be to initially stabilise the level of obesity in the population, reduce the incidence of new cases and then, in time, to reduce the overall prevalence of obesity.[1] This would mean not only targeting those individuals at risk of obesity[2] but, in light of the health benefits of maintaining a healthy weight, making the prevention and management of obesity a priority for all.[3]

Such an approach would view children as a particularly important target, as they are at a time in their lives in which small changes are effective.[4,5] Plus the low rate of obesity in every new birth cohort is easier to maintain than to decrease in later life. However, changing the prevalence rates of early-childhood obesity will, in the short term, have little influence on overall prevalence in the population.[5,6] Population prevention interventions must, therefore, target all age groups, influencing behaviour throughout the life-course.[5,7]

This aim for the prevention of obesity calls for change at all levels, not just for individuals but also for the organisations which influence them.[6] This should lead to multidisciplinary approaches[8] which encourage behaviour change[9] and establish new social norms[10] through the creation of supportive environments.[11]

## Population approach

As the current obesity epidemic is the result of a large number of interacting influences it must be tackled from multiple angles[2] through a population-oriented approach.[12,13] This is done by striking a better balance between 'individual and population-wide approaches'[13] by combining population-based measures and local 'settings-based' approaches.[14] A comprehensive long-term strategy must act to create an environment that supports and facilitates healthy choices and encourages individuals to desire, seek and make different choices, recognising that decisions and behaviours are 'cued' by the behaviours of others.[6] Population-level approaches include policy and environmental change[3,13,15] along with regulatory and fiscal measures[2] implemented through a multisectoral and multistakeholder programme.[2,5,13]

Throughout this chapter we discuss population prevention approaches to obesity by focusing on four keys areas:[3,13,16]

1. Targeting, development and monitoring.
2. Multifactorial approach.
3. Involvement of numerous stakeholders.
4. The targeting of all settings.

## Targeting, development and monitoring
### Targeting

The International Obesity Taskforce (IOTF) advise that targeted outcomes are important for obesity prevention, describing two types: impact and process, both of which may take years to achieve.[17] Impact outcomes refer to the ultimate targets of obesity-prevention programmes, relating to the level of obesity in a population.[17] These could include a target to shift the BMI distribution of the population and lower the population mean.[2] Process outcomes relate to the processes that will lead to these impact outcomes, such as changes in food intake and physical activity patterns amongst the population.[17] However, although many governments set targets to combat obesity in health policies, the use of these can be contentious as it is thought that these can lead to 'gaming', decrease staff morale and encourage the disproportionate diversion of resources.[18,19] Indeed, in some countries early targets that were set have been abandoned or updated.[19]

As well as targeting the desired outcomes of any intervention, targeting the factors an intervention must overcome is also important.[20] Due to the numerous influences on obesity this can be challenging and the WHO describe the use of ANGELO (analysis grid for elements linked to obesity), developed for scanning environments for obesogenic barriers,[21] suggesting that this provides the necessary structure for conceptualising the multitude of factors that contribute to obesity.[13] The ANGELO process fits within the overall health promotion process by undertaking a situation analysis, setting priorities for action, gaining consensus on an action plan and building community capacity by increasing skills, knowledge and ownership through five key areas:[13,21]

1. Community engagement.
2. Gathering intelligence.

3. Updating stakeholders.
4. Scoring priority elements.
5. Forming the action plan.

## Development

Any course of action taken to prevent obesity should be evidence-based. However, as knowledge on appropriate public health obesity prevention interventions is limited[5,22] the 'best evidence available' should be used, as distinct from the 'best evidence possible'.[23,24] This is because evidence-based medicine type criteria are too narrow for public health purposes, as they lead to the reliance on randomised controlled trials (RCT) as the optimal quality standard, encouraging the view that any other type of evidence is less worthwhile.[25] For public health purposes, however, RCT evidence is often inappropriate, unachievable, or irrelevant because the RCT requirement to manipulate a single, or limited set of variables may be too artificial or unrealistic (or unethical) for the complex systems.[24] Following best evidence possible will allow more immediate action to be taken, leading to incremental change of interventions through the concept of better practice rather than 'best practice'.[6] With this in mind evidence of effectiveness is not the only guide[26] with 'practice-based evidence'[27] used over 'evidence-based practice'[24] and decision makers considering implementation issues including

feasibility, sustainability, effects on equity and cost-effectiveness.[5,24]

Cost-effectiveness in particular is becoming an increasingly important factor in decision making in the implementation of prevention programmes, with cost limitations a consideration in all countries.[5,13] The assessment of cost effectiveness can be done in a number of ways, with the WHO describing ACE-Obesity (assessing the cost-effectiveness of obesity interventions)[28] as a method by which to do this.[13] To help with cost-effectiveness, as well as other implementation issues, interventions can be developed which are embedded into already on-going programmes and operating systems, avoiding the costly initial implementation of new stand-alone interventions.[22]

## Monitoring

Evaluation and monitoring is an essential tool in any programme. It can provide information on many aspects of the programme as well as providing feedback to allow improvements to be made. It is also thought that monitoring can acknowledge the efforts of those involved in any intervention as well as documenting experience gained from the project, such that it can be shared with others.[17]

The WHO describes three types of indicators which can be used in monitoring obesity prevention programmes:[13,29]

1. Process indicators used to measure progress and quality of the implementation. These relate to input, focusing on how something has been done and include indicators such as human and financial resources.
2. Output indicators used to assess the outputs or products, such as that from supportive programmes, environments and policies.
3. Outcome indicators used to measure the ultimate outcomes of an action. These can include impact and process outcomes and can be short term such as increased knowledge; intermediate such as a change in behaviour; or long term such as a reduction in the prevalence.

Evaluation should commence from the beginning of any intervention and continue throughout it. It should be built into each action and programme and incorporated into any budget. For countries with limited resources, intermediate-term process evaluation may be more feasible than long-term outcome evaluation, which can be costly and complex.[17] To avoid extra costs or resources it may be possible to utilise monitoring activities and databases that are already established at the local, national and international levels such as national surveys and data collection programmes.[13] The WHO also suggest the use of health impact assessment (HIA) in examining the impact of all policies on health outcomes.[13]

> ## ! Thinking points
>
> 1. When targeting all individuals in a population, can we consider implementing one overarching intervention?
> 2. What will influence which outcome measures should be targeted when developing a population prevention programme?
> 3. What are the pros and cons of evidence-based medicine in population obesity prevention programmes?
> 4. What are the most important factors to consider in the monitoring of population approaches to combat obesity?

## Multifactorial approach

A population-level prevention programme must be multifaceted and include intervention at a number of levels. In Chapter 5, some of the small-scale interventions are discussed, in particular as part of a health services approach to tackling obesity. In this section we discuss macro-level interventions which can be implemented with the view of influencing the whole population, at the centre of which is an overarching policy.

## Policy

Many countries recognise the important role of national policies in preventing obesity, including policies related to food and physical activity, with most acknowledging the central role of an environmental approach to improving health.[13] However, the detail and implementation of these policies differs widely between countries[30] with some describing a 'policy cacophony' in which the 'noise is drowning out the symphony of effort'[19,31] making the task of obesity prevention appear difficult.[5] Additionally the creation and implementation of policies can be challenging, due to the complexity of obesity causation, the lack of evidence on effective intervention along with political pressures from the private sector and other agencies.[19] The making of public health policy involves competing interests with competing demands being placed upon policy-makers and it is, therefore, an inherently political process, based on competing human values, interests and beliefs.[32,33] The viability of government policies isn't just a matter of what works in theory, but what works in a manner that society finds acceptable.[31]

Evidence does show that prevention policies, particularly focused on improving diets and activity,[2,34] could have a major impact on population health and prove to be cost-effective.[2] Investment in policies focused on obesity prevention, along with investment in the capability to deliver such policies, could have benefits not only in major reductions in health-related costs, but also in broader societal benefits arising from improved well-being and quality of life.[31] Any policy, however, in order

to be successful depends on high-level political commitment, full involvement of all government sectors and effective coordination[30] with guidance on the principles for the development of national policy to prevent obesity provided by organisations such as the WHO.[14]

If new policies are to be effective, they must embrace the policy remit of numerous government departments and other important sectors, such as the food industry, in an integrated fashion. Although the repercussions of obesity mainly burden the health system, ministries outside health, such as finance, education, agriculture, transportation and urban planning, arguably have the greatest influence in creating environments conducive to prevention,[5] including agricultural policies discussed in Chapter 4. If health policies are developed in isolation from these influential ministries, there is a very high risk that positive action in one area might be undermined by well-intentioned but opposing forces in another.[6] For example, changes to dietary patterns may impact on the production and processing of food, which may impact on the climate if these foods require importation or greater land use in production.

Additionally action through alignment with other major policy issues is critical in order to maximise the engagement of a broad range of stakeholders. Policies in other departments can act to reduce the prevalence of obesity through actions motivated by other policy priorities. For example, policies to reduce carbon emissions to mitigate climate change, such as increasing the cyclability and walkability of the built environment, have the potential to have a direct impact on the prevalence of obesity. Indeed policies relating to climate change and health inequalities were identified as particularly critical partners in the development of a strategy to tackle obesity.[35–38]

## Information

The WHO describe that a key role for governments in combating obesity is to provide 'accurate and balanced information' to the general population, regarding diet and nutrition as well as physical activity.[39] Many governments provide guidance on obesity-related health behaviours through promotional messages such as '5 a Day' in the UK, USA and New Zealand; 'Go for 2 and 5' in Australia and 'Mix it up!' in Canada; along with information on energy and dietary balance as well as physical activity guidelines. However, there is still a need to effectively disseminate this information on the subject to have any impact, whilst there is still scope for improving the information-base upon which individuals make their dietary choices.[34]

Providing information to consumers on the food available to them is seen as a common way to influence choice.[34]

Almost all food policies recommend food labelling as an important provision of this type of information, in particular front-of-pack labelling,[5] with this type of information thought to impact on dietary choices.[34,40–42] Such front-of-pack labelling includes the 'traffic-light system' used in the United Kingdom since 2005. These labels, now accompanying the majority of processed foods in the UK, have been found to reduce confusion and help consumers make healthier choices, as well as being thought to encourage manufacturers to reformulate products to improve their nutritional quality.[43] However, although the UK Food Standards Agency has recommended that a traffic light front-of-pack labelling system should be adopted by all food manufacturers[19] this has not occurred universally and some manufacturers have developed their own forms of label. The existence of multiple labelling systems has created inconsistency in the provision of consumer information[19] along with uncontrolled industry-produced health claims which can give a product a halo effect, potentially discouraging consumers from seeking further nutrition information, encouraging them to buy the product and to consume more of it.[13] Proposals are in place for a standardised approach to labelling, although this is still seen to be voluntary and some suggest that legislation may be required to overcome some of the weaknesses of this approach.[19,44] Labelling can also potentially be extended to a number of areas such as restaurants, cinemas and in advertising.[45] However, labelling has been heavily contested by the food industry, so compulsory implementation is politically difficult.[5]

## Fiscal intervention

Fiscal interventions are another means by which governments can influence choice. This occurs through raising prices on unhealthy behaviours and/or decreasing the cost on healthy ones.[34] A classic example of a fiscal intervention is taxation, with studies of tax and price policies applied to tobacco and alcohol products in many countries providing persuasive evidence of their effects on decreasing consumption.[34] Such policies may serve as a model for lowering consumption of foods high in saturated fats and other energy-dense foods.[13] Indeed tax exemptions and subsidies are already widely used in agriculture and food markets, whilst differential taxation of food products is relatively common with value-added or sales taxes often applied at different rates to different types of products.[34,46] A proposed intervention for reducing the consumption of energy-dense and high-fat drinks and foods is to implement a 'sin' or 'junk food' tax.[43,47] Such taxes may have the effect of raising prices above some consumers' willingness to pay, leading them to reduce or stop consumption of the undesirable product. However, depending on the elasticity of the demand for the taxed

product, consumers will either end up bearing an extra financial burden, or changing the mix of products they consume in ways that can be difficult to identify.[34] Some consumers may respond by reducing their consumption of other goods, including healthy ones, in order to pay for the more expensive unhealthy goods, thus defeating the purpose of the tax. Others may seek substitutes for the taxed product, which might be as unhealthy as those originally consumed. To counter this, a combination of increased prices in the form of taxes for nutrients such as fat, saturated fat and sugar could be implemented alongside subsidies on healthy foods with any policies that raise the prices of particular foods without a complementary subsidy viewed by some as inequitable.[13,45,48] In fact a dedicated junk food tax may generate large revenues that could then be used to subsidise these healthy food prices or to fund obesity-prevention programmes.[13,43,47,49]

Supporters of such an approach suggest that these taxes may prove to be cost-effective as benefits accrue to the entire population and the cost of implementation is relatively low.[5] Opponents of an unhealthy food tax, however, have identified several potential barriers, including the relative inelasticity of unhealthy food consumption (i.e. a cost increase may not create a substantial reduction in consumption); a potential shift in demand to other non-taxed energy-dense foods; and the difficulty in defining which foods should be taxed. It has also been suggested that such taxes have a disproportionately negative effect on lower socioeconomic classes, which are typically more dependent on fast foods for their nutrition.[43,50] Lastly, public opposition to such taxes may be substantial.[43]

There are also fiscal interventions which relate to the promotion of physical activity. For example, the supply of 'sporting services' or sports goods[45] can be made exempt from value-added tax. The construction of sports facilities may also avoid value-added tax if not for profit; however, this is a complex and fact-dependent area of law that may prove difficult to navigate for community activity providers.[51] A public investment in a new form of transportation such as bikes in major cities, or a programme of subsidies to make public transportation more convenient and less expensive[34] or a focus on the restriction of automated traffic[51] may encourage more active travel. However, many of these interventions are implemented at a potentially high cost.[34]

## Legislation

The law is recognised as a powerful tool to address some of the structural determinants of chronic disease, including obesogenic environments.[51] Many of the elements of an environment are shaped by an overarching regulatory framework composed of a range of laws and measures found at a number of

levels.[49,51] Indeed in many countries it is not only national but also local legislation which can have a major influence on the built environment and community,[51,52] such as the control of licences for fast-food restaurants.[51] Law can influence unhealthy behaviour in a number of ways. In light of the perceived failings of self-regulation by the food industry[51,53,54] many suggest that regulation is effective in directly prohibiting harmful behaviours and de-normalising unhealthy choices, such as reducing smoking in enclosed public areas.[51,55] Legislation can spread to influence every setting that the law can apply to, including the school environment, the built environment, community facilities and point-of-sale environments, as well as considering areas of food production and processing.[51,55,56] Such regulation can also influence areas which reach the majority of individuals in a population such as restrictions on the advertising of certain foods to children, mostly carried out on television, implemented in a number of countries.[34,51] These can be extended as far as banning certain foods such as that implemented to ban trans-fats in Denmark and New York City.[57]

Such legislative interventions place responsibility at the societal and population levels and focus on modifiable environmental contributors[43,49,58] as well as strengthening stakeholders' participation by removing a dependence on voluntary participation.[13]

## Stakeholders

Involving multiple stakeholders and encouraging them to support the implementation of comprehensive long-term strategies, is a crucial part of developing population-level strategies.[13,34,59] This can be challenging as not all stakeholders commit to health.[13] There are a number of stakeholders recognised which would have a part to play in obesity prevention, including:[6]

1. National governments/leaders.
2. Local governments/leaders.
3. International agencies.
4. Health and social services.
5. Private sector.
6. Media.
7. Academia.
8. Non-governmental organisations (NGOs).

### National government

A population obesity prevention approach requires the lead from national government[6] through the substantial involvement and investment at all levels.[45] Only national guidance, along with funding, can ensure effectiveness and sustainability of action at a population level[14] and a strong policy from government agency allows the effective involvement of many stakeholders.[13]

Governments are recognised as the most important actors in reversing the obesity epidemic.[5] We look to governments to protect public welfare through a combination of a number of approaches including regulation, taxes, or education.[34] Safeguarding public health is a fundamental responsibility of governments and they need to provide leadership and formulate, monitor and evaluate comprehensive policies.[13] The government has a role in managing the process of developing, implementing and monitoring a national strategy to prevent obesity, with all the ministries and sectors involved in implementation also involved in developing the strategy.[13]

### Local government

Local government is also important in any population-level approach. Strategic action must be coherent, with local strategies reflecting local conditions, needs and aspirations. Any national strategy must, therefore, provide clear definitions for the role of local government.[6] Local governments are important as they have a role in creating supportive environments for health behaviours.[16,33] This includes controlling urban development and planning, managing a number of local settings such as schools, supporting local markets that sustain local agriculture and horticulture and setting local economic priorities.[13] These local authorities should then work with local partners, such as industry and voluntary organisations in implementing a prevention approach.[3]

### Health and social services

Health and social services can play an important role in the population prevention of obesity beyond clinical interventions discussed in Chapter 5. They can work in partnerships with local authorities to encourage community networks in support of health promotion.[13] They can also act as providers of information for things such as healthy eating, physical activity and in the promotion of practices such as breastfeeding.[13] Health services can also help in targeting individuals and play a role in monitoring BMI change through regular measurements, whilst some behaviour change interventions that form one part of a multifaceted population approach can be based in general practice[60] such as promoting physical activity.[61,62]

### International agencies

There are a number of international agencies which can be involved in action to prevent obesity. These include those that affect public health such as the United Nations (UN), the WHO and associated agencies.[5] Political, economic and trade-related multi-national bodies also have a profound effect on obesity prevalence, including the World Trade Organisation, the World Bank, International Monetary Fund and European Union.[5] Agencies such as the WHO also produce and disseminate a number of tools which can assist Member States and associated stakeholders in implementing strategies to prevent obesity[13] as well as developing global strategies to combat obesity-related behaviours.[29]

### Private sector

The private sector plays an increasingly influential role in shaping the environments we live in, as well as developing accepted social norms through marketing and advertising. On top of this they can influence policy through funds and lobbying. Active support from this sector would, therefore, be helpful in developing a population approach to prevent obesity.[5] However, many such stakeholders, with considerable influence over food, don't recognise their potential contribution and are of the opinion that they serve different clients,[13] in particular their shareholders, which has led some to reject the promotion of healthier products.[57] Although some from the private sector have engaged in health promotion, in response to the demand of consumers, such as the development of a health and well-being industry, this appears to be mostly confined to certain population groups, in particular those that are of least risk.[34,63,64] An option, therefore, is to encourage companies to adopt a more healthful approach through government regulation, although governments are often reluctant to do this due to the complexity of the regulatory process, the potential costs and the possible confrontation with industry.[34]

## Media

The media play a major role in information dissemination, informal education and reflecting and shaping public attitudes.[6] It can reach vast audiences rapidly and directly.[34] The media can, therefore, be utilised in public health programmes and should be controlled and regulated in influences such as the advertising of unhealthy products and behaviour. This is particularly important when directed at children, who do not distinguish advertising from other forms of programming.[45] There is an increasing interest in using advertising techniques for socially beneficial purposes, referred to as social marketing.[13] However, research on social marketing suggests that it is unlikely that the type of public information campaigns that urge people to avoid certain foods and to exercise more frequently will be enough to adequately address the problem of obesity[65–67] and interventions must go beyond information campaigns to encompass environmental change.

## Other stakeholders

Non-governmental organisations, civil society and academia can all play a role through the advocacy and development of guidance and policies; the dissemination and evaluation of practice; the documentation and monitoring of approaches and stakeholder roles; as well as raising awareness and providing information on obesity prevention.[14] Such stakeholders should be involved at the early stages of any intervention.

---

**! Thinking points**

1. Why is it crucial to have a lead from government in any population obesity prevention programme?
2. What role can international agencies play in a national obesity programme?
3. What are the challenges to working with the private sector in obesity prevention?
4. Social marketing is a popular approach with governments to influence behaviour despite the lack of evidence of its effectiveness; why could this be?

---

## Settings

As obesity is a population-wide problem, public health interventions should target all settings. Some of the more important settings which should be included in such an approach are:

## Schools

Schools and early years settings are key environments through which to reach children. Although on their own the impact of schools may be limited, it will be very difficult to achieve any success in a population approach to obesity without their support. In general a 'whole school' approach to health, both diet and physical activity, leading to supportive environments within schools is thought to be the most effective.[31,68,69] These whole school approaches carry health promotion messages in all aspects of school life not just through education in the classroom.[3,22] National and local regulation can help schools by implementing interventions that promote healthful behaviours, such as controlling the sale of competitive foods, and creating nutritional guidelines and regulations; as well as providing funding for any changes schools are required to implement.[3,16,45]

## Work place

Although the policy and sociocultural environment in the work place is an important determinant of behaviour there is a consideration that to date, in some countries, the potential for using workplaces for obesity prevention has not been fully exploited.[19] Certainly employers can influence both diet and activity behaviour through food available, parking and transport policies and by encouraging active recreation or discounted leisure facility costs.[3] Although employers can be encouraged to do this through tax incentives and company regulation, it remains unclear whether or not corporate incentives are a viable policy option to fight the obesity epidemic.[43]

## Communities

The community environment can be modified to be less obesogenic through both regulation of the environment and urban design, an inter-disciplinary subject that unites all the built environment professions, including urban planning, landscape architecture, architecture, civil and municipal engineering.[43] Indeed although urbanisation has traditionally been linked to ill health, including obesity, urbanisation may very well be part of the solution if urban design and local governance are geared towards promoting active and nutritious cities.[14]

Local authorities have control over many of the environmental determinants of obesity, including planning control of physical urban development.[51] This could lead to the provision of incentives for communities to develop safe and accessible activity environments and facilities.[13,45] Additionally in some instances local governance has the power of regulation for licences for fast-food restaurants, which enables them to control both the location and density of these, controlling proximity to certain key settings such as schools.[51,70] In England the 'Healthy Towns' initiative recognised the role of local environments by encouraging the provision of environments which encouraged physical activity.[19,45]

Indeed community settings offer opportunities to reach various individuals and groups at the local level[13] and are seen as a necessary complement to the implementation of macro-level policies. Members of a community share cultural or ethnic backgrounds and are exposed to the same environmental determinants. All community programmes should, therefore, address the concerns of local people from the outset[3,34] gathering information about the community and tracking progress over time.[16]

A number of community interventions have produced impressive results in reducing lifestyle risk factors, such as the 'North Karelia Project' in Eastern Finland.[71,72] Two key factors in this success are the ability of interventions to generate sustained changes in people's behaviours, and the extent to which individuals targeted by interventions respond.[2] A number of organisations, including the CDC and the WHO, have published guidance on implementing community strategies to encourage and support healthy eating and active living.[14,16] An example of a community-wide obesity prevention programme is EPODE (see the EPODE Case Study in Box 6.1).

---

### Box 6.1 Case study: EPODE

Ensemble, Prévenons l'Obésité Des Enfants (EPODE) translated as '*Together Let's Prevent Childhood Obesity*' targets children aged 0 to 12 years along with their families and is thought to be the largest global childhood obesity prevention programme.[73] EPODE was first launched in 2004 in ten French pilot communities, in line with official French guidelines on diet and physical activity[74] and has since expanded to more than 500 communities worldwide.[73] Early evaluation of the EPODE methodology suggests encouraging results[73,75] through a reduction of the prevalence of being overweight or obese.[34,76,77] In France, the project is funded at the national level by the private sector and at the local level by public funds; however, local authorities are free to set up their own private–public partnerships to secure additional funding, as long as the prescribed rules are followed.[14]

EPODE is a multi-stakeholder, capacity-building approach which allows communities to implement effective and sustainable strategies to prevent childhood obesity.[14] Involvement of multiple stakeholders occurs at a central level (ministries, health groups, non-governmental organisations [NGOs] and private partners) and a local level (political leaders, health professionals, families, teachers, local NGOs and the local business community).[73] At the central level, a coordination team uses social marketing and organisational techniques in training and coaching a local project manager nominated in each EPODE community by the local authorities. The local project manager is also provided with tools to mobilise local stakeholders through a local steering committee and local networks. The added value of the methodology is to mobilise stakeholders at all levels across the public and the private sectors.[73] EPODE methodology has four critical 'pillars':

*Continued*

1. Political commitment at central and local levels.
2. Resources to fund central support services and evaluation, as well as contributions from local organisations to fund local implementation.
3. Support services to plan, coordinate, and provide aspects of the intervention including the social marketing, communication and support services for community practitioners and leaders.
4. Evidence from a wide variety of sources used to inform delivery of EPODE and to evaluate process, impact and outcomes of the EPODE programme.[73]

### Thinking points

1. Is health promotion a responsibility of schools?
2. What reasons could there be that the work place is a setting which has not been fully exploited in preventing obesity?
3. How can urbanisation be seen as both a potential cause and a preventative factor for obesity?
4. What are the challenges to implementing successful community interventions in other communities or countries?

### Summary points

- A population approach to prevent obesity should target all individuals and change at all levels.
- Programmes must clearly target desired outcomes which can be related to either impacts or processes.
- In a population approach the best evidence available can be used in developing programmes, as distinct from the best evidence possible.
- Evaluation and monitoring should commence from the beginning of any intervention and continue throughout it by being built into each action and programme as well as being budgeted for.
- A population-level prevention programme must be multifaceted and include intervention at a number of levels.
- National and local policy plays a central role in any population-level prevention programme.
- Successful policy requires high-level political commitment, full involvement of all government sectors and effective coordination.
- A key role for governments in combating obesity is to provide accurate and balanced information to the general population.

*Continued*

- Fiscal interventions should consider issues of inequity and the balance between taxation and subsidy to encourage healthy behaviours.
- Many of the elements of an environment are shaped by an overarching regulatory framework composed of a range of laws and measures found at a number of levels.
- Involving multiple stakeholders and encouraging them to support the implementation of comprehensive long-term strategies, is a crucial part of developing population-level strategies.
- A population obesity prevention approach requires the lead from government through the substantial involvement of and investment at all levels.
- Although active support from the private sector is helpful in developing a population approach to prevent obesity, they often don't recognise their potential contribution and are of the opinion that they serve different clients.
- The media can be utilised in public health programmes and should be controlled and regulated in influences such as the advertising of unhealthy products and behaviour.
- There are a number of key settings which should be targeted by a population-level obesity prevention programme; these include schools and places of work.
- Community settings offer opportunities to reach various individuals and groups at the local level, with a number of community interventions found to impact on reducing lifestyle risk factors.

## Web pages and resources

Association for the Study of Obesity (ASO) factsheets.
www.aso.org.uk/useful-resources/obesity-fact-sheets/.
National Schools Board Association (NSBA) – Preventing Childhood Obesity.
www.nsba.org/Board-Leadership/SchoolHealth/obesity-and-schools.
CDC's LEAN *Works!* – A Workplace Obesity Prevention Program.
www.cdc.gov/leanworks/.
EPODE international network.
www.epode-international-network.com/.

## Further reading

1. WHO. Population Based Prevention Strategies for Childhood Obesity. Geneva: World Health Organization; 2010.
   http://www.who.int/dietphysicalactivity/childhood/child-obesity-eng.pdf.
   *This report presents a set of guiding principles for childhood obesity policy and programme development and examples of areas for action, along with summaries of presentations on country experiences in prevention interventions.*
2. Gortmaker, et al. Changing the future of obesity: science, policy, and action. Lancet 2011;378:838–47.
   http://www.thelancet.com/journals/lancet/article/PIIS0140-6736%2811%2960815-5/abstract.
   *This report presents findings from evidence on obesity interventions, outlines a strategy for the prevention of obesity that builds on this growing science and specifically links evidence for effectiveness and cost with implementation feasibility and other concerns of policy makers.*

3. Cecchini M, Sassi F. Tackling obesity requires efficient government policies. Isr J Health Policy Res 2012;1:18.
http://www.ncbi.nlm.nih.gov/pmc/articles/PMC3424968/pdf/2045-4015-1-18.pdf.

*A short commentary piece which summarises reasoning for government-lead national and community-level interventions to prevent obesity at a population level.*

*To view the full reference list for the book, click here http://dx.doi.org/10.1016/ B978-0-7020-4634-6.00006-6

# References

A full list of references can be accessed online at: http://evolve.
elsevier.com/

## Chapter 1

[1] WHO. Obesity: preventing and managing the global epidemic. Report of a WHO consultation. World Health Organ Tech Rep Ser 2000;894:i–xii,1–253.

[2] Bray GA, Bouchard C, James WPT. Handbook of obesity: etiology and pathophysiology. CRC Press; 2003.

[9] Nihiser AJ, Lee SM, Wechsler H, et al. Body mass index measurement in schools. J Sch Health 2007;77:651–71; quiz 722–724.

[14] IC. National Child Measurement Programme: England, 2009/10 school year. Leeds: The Information Centre for Health and Social Care; 2010.

[17] CGOU. Healthy Weight, Healthy Lives: National Child Measurement Programme Guidance for Primary Care Trusts 2009/10. London: Cross Government Obesity Unit; 2009.

[20] Merrill RM, Richardson JS. Validity of self-reported height, weight, and body mass index: findings from the National Health and Nutrition Examination Survey, 2001–2006. Prev Chronic Dis 2009;6:A121.

[21] Stommel M, Schoenborn CA. Accuracy and usefulness of BMI measures based on self-reported weight and height: findings from the NHANES & NHIS 2001–2006. BMC Public Health 2009;9:421.

[22] Krul AJ, Daanen HAM, Choi H. Self-reported and measured weight, height and body mass index (BMI) in Italy, the Netherlands and North America. Eur J Public Health 2011;21:414–9.

[23] Rowland ML. Self-reported weight and height. Am J Clin Nutr 1990;52:1125–33.

[37] NHMRC. Clinical practice guidelines for the management of overweight and obesity in adults. National Health & Medical Research Council; 2003a.

[38] NICE. Obesity: Guidance on the prevention, identification, assessment and management of overweight and obesity in adults and children (CG 43). (Guidance/Clinical Guidelines). London: National Institute for Health and Clinical Excellence; 2006.

[39] NIH. Clinical guidelines on the identification, evaluation, and treatment of overweight and obesity in adults: the evidence report. National Institutes of Health, National Heart, Lung, and Blood Institute; 1998.

[41] Forbes GB, Halloran E. The adult decline in lean body mass. Hum Biol 1976;48:161–73.

[42] Rolland-Cachera MF, Cole TJ, Sempé M, et al. Body Mass Index variations: centiles from birth to 87 years. Eur J Clin Nutr 1991;45:13–21.

[43] Swinburn BA, Craig PL, Daniel R, et al. Body composition differences between Polynesians and Caucasians assessed by bioelectrical impedance. Int J Obes Relat Metab Disord 1996;20:889–94.

[44] Reilly JJ, Methven E, Dowell ZCM, et al. Health consequences of obesity. Arch Dis Child 2003;88.

[47] Sardinha LB, Lohman TG, Teixeira PJ, et al. Comparison of air displacement plethysmography with dual-energy X-ray

# References

absorptiometry and 3 field methods for estimating body composition in middle-aged men. Am J Clin Nutr 1998;68:786–93.

[48] Browning LM, Mugridge O, Dixon AK, et al. Measuring abdominal adipose tissue: comparison of simpler methods with MRI. Obes Facts 2011;4:9–15.

[61] Lee CMY, Huxley RR, Wildman RP, et al. Indices of abdominal obesity are better discriminators of cardiovascular risk factors than BMI: a meta-analysis. J Clin Epidemiol 2008;61:646–53.

[62] NOO. Measures of central adiposity as an indicator of obesity. Oxford: National Obesity Observatory; 2009.

[70] Valdez R, Seidell JC, Ahn YI, et al. A new index of abdominal adiposity as an indicator of risk for cardiovascular disease. A cross-population study. Int J Obes Relat Metab Disord 1993;17:77–82.

[72] McCarthy HD, Ashwell M. A study of central fatness using waist-to-height ratios in UK children and adolescents over two decades supports the simple message –'keep your waist circumference to less than half your height'. Int J Obes (Lond) 2006;30:988–92.

[75] NHMRC. Clinical Practice Guidelines for the Management of Overweight and Obesity in Children and Adolescents. National Health & Medical Research Council; 2003b.

[76] Browning LM, Mugridge O, Chatfield MD, et al. Validity of a new abdominal bioelectrical impedance device to measure abdominal and visceral fat: comparison with MRI. Obesity (Silver Spring) 2010;18:2385–91.

[78] Brodie D, Moscrip H, Hutcheon R. Body Composition Measurement: A Review of Hydrodensitometry, Anthropometry, and Impedance Methods. Nutrition 1998;14:296–310.

[80] Medeiros-Neto G, Halpern A, Bouchard C. Progress in obesity research: 9. John Libbey Eurotext, 2003.

[81] Kopelman PG, Caterson ID, Dietz WH. Clinical Obesity in Adults and Children. John Wiley and Sons; 2009.

[83] Lee RE, Booth KM, Reese-Smith JY, et al. The Physical Activity Resource Assessment (PARA) instrument: Evaluating

features, amenities and incivilities of physical activity resources in urban neighbourhoods. Int J Behav Nutr Phys Act 2005;2:13.

[84] Snijder MB, Visser M, Dekker JM, et al. The prediction of visceral fat by dual-energy X-ray absorptiometry in the elderly: a comparison with computed tomography and anthropometry. Int J Obes Relat Metab Disord 2002;26:984–93.

[85] Van der Kooy K, Seidell JC. Techniques for the measurement of visceral fat: a practical guide. Int J Obes Relat Metab Disord 1993;17:187–96.

[87] Treleaven, Wells JCK. 3D body scanning and healthcare applications. Computer 2007;40:28–34.

[88] Wells JCK, Ruto A, Treleaven P. Whole-body three-dimensional photonic scanning: a new technique for obesity research and clinical practice. Int J Obes (Lond) 2008;32:232–8.

[89] Di Lorenzo N, Servidio M, Di Renzo L, et al. Is Digital Image Plethysmographic (DIP) Acquisition a Valid New Tool for Preoperative Body Composition Assessment? A Validation by Dual-energy X-ray Absorptiometry. Obesity Surgery 2006;16:560–6.

[97] Häger A, Sjöstrm L, Arvidsson B, et al. Body fat and adipose tissue cellularity in infants: a longitudinal study. Metab Clin Exp 1977;26:607–14.

[98] Knittle JL, Timmers K, Ginsberg-Fellner F, et al. The growth of adipose tissue in children and adolescents. Cross-sectional and longitudinal studies of adipose cell number and size. J Clin Invest 1979;63:239–46.

[99] Rolland-Cachera M, Deheeger M, Bellisle F, et al. Adiposity rebound in children: a simple indicator for predicting obesity. Am J Clin Nutr 1984;39:129–35.

[100] Taylor RW, Grant AM, Goulding A, et al. Early adiposity rebound: review of papers linking this to subsequent obesity in children and adults. Curr Opin Clin Nutr Metab Care 2005;8:607–12.

[102] Williams SM. Weight and Height Growth Rate and the Timing of Adiposity Rebound. Obesity 2005;13:1123–30.

[107] Cole TJ. Children grow and horses race: is the adiposity rebound a critical period for later obesity? BMC Pediatr 2004;4:6.

## Chapter 2

[1] NHS IC. Health Survey for England – 2010: Trend tables. [WWW Document]. URL http://www.hscic.gov.uk/pubs/hse10trends; 2012a [accessed 06.06.12].

[2] NHS IC. National Child Measurement Programme: England, 2010/11 school year [WWW Document]. URL http://www.ic.nhs.uk/ncmp; 2012 [accessed 06.06.12].

[3] Scottish Executive, S.A.H. Datasets [WWW Document]. URL www.scotland.gov.uk/Topics/Statistics/Browse/Health/scottish-health-survey/SHeSDatasets; 2010 [accessed 06.06.12].

[4] Welsh Government. Welsh Health Survey: Results. [WWW Document]. URL http://wales.gov.uk/topics/statistics/theme/health/health-survey/results/?lang=en; 2012 [accessed 06.06.12].

[5] Northern Ireland Statistics and Research Agency. Northern Ireland Health and Social WellBeing Survey 2005/06. [WWW Document]. URL www.csu.nisra.gov.uk/survey.asp5.htm; 2007 [accessed 06.06.12].

[6] Northern Ireland Department of Health, S.S. and P.S. 15 November 2011 – Health Survey Northern Ireland: first results from the 2010/11 survey | Northern Ireland Executive. [WWW Document]. URL http://www.northernireland.gov.uk/index/media-centre/news-departments/news-dhssps/news-dhssps-151111-health-survey-northern.htm; 2011 [accessed 06.06.12].

[8] Irish Universities Nutrition Alliance. National Teen's Food Survey. Cork: University College Cork; 2008.

[9] Ogden CL, Carroll MD, Kit BK, et al. Prevalence of obesity in the United States, 2009–2010. NCHS data brief, no 82. Hyattsville, MD: National Center for Health Statistics; 2012.

[11] Government of Canada, S.C. Canadian Health Measures Survey (CHMS). [WWW Document]. URL www.statcan.gc.ca/imdb-bmdi/5071-eng.htm; 2009 [accessed 06.06.12].

[12] Australian Bureau of Statistics. National Health Survey 2007–8: Summary of Results. Canberra: Australian Bureau of Statistics; 2009.

[13] Ministry of Health. The Health of New Zealand Adults 2011/12: Key findings of the New Zealand Health Survey. Wellington: Ministry of Health; 2012.

[21] Wang YC, McPherson K, Marsh T, et al. Health and economic burden of the projected obesity trends in the USA and the UK. Lancet 2011;378:815–25.

[23] Wardle J, Brodersen NH, Cole TJ, et al. Development of adiposity in adolescence: five year longitudinal study of an ethnically and socioeconomically diverse sample of young people in Britain. BMJ 2006;332:1130–5.

[24] Saxena S, Ambler G, Cole T, et al. Ethnic group differences in overweight and obese children and young people in England: cross sectional survey. Arch Dis Child 2004;89:30–6.

[39] Shaw NJ, Crabtree NJ, Kibirige MS, et al. Ethnic and gender differences in body fat in British schoolchildren as measured by DXA. Arch Dis Child 2007;92:872–5.

[40] Jebb SA, Rennie KL, Cole TJ. Prevalence of overweight and obesity among young people in Great Britain. Public Health Nutr 2004;7:461–5.

[41] Rona RJ, Chinn S. National Study of Health and Growth: social and biological factors associated with weight-for-height and triceps skinfold of children from ethnic groups in England. Ann Hum Biol 1987;14:231–48.

[55] Marmot M, Allen J, Goldblatt P, et al. Fair Society, Healthy Lives: Strategic Review of Health Inequalities in England post-2010, The Marmot Review. London: University College; 2010.

[56] Stamatakis E, Wardle J, Cole TJ. Childhood obesity and overweight prevalence trends in England: evidence for growing socioeconomic disparities. Int J Obes 2009;34:41–7.

[58] Stafford M, Brunner EJ, Head J, et al. Deprivation and the Development of Obesity: A Multilevel, Longitudinal Study in England. Am J Prev Med 2010;39:130–9.

[60] Ogden C, Lamb M, Carroll M, et al. Obesity and socioeconomic status in adults: United States 1988–1994 and 2005–2008. NCHS data brief no 50. Hyattsville, MD: National Center for Health Statistics; 2010.

# Chapter 3

[3] Kava R, Ross G, Whelan E. Obesity and its Health Effects. New York: American Council on Science and Health; 2008.

[4] Peeters A, Barendregt JJ, Willekens F, et al. Obesity in adulthood and its consequences for life expectancy: a life-table analysis. Ann Intern Med 2003;138:24–32.

[5] WHO. The Challenge of obesity in the WHO European Region and the strategies for response. Denmark: WHO Regional Office for Europe; 2007.

[6] Higdon JV, Frei B. Obesity and Oxidative Stress A Direct Link to CVD? Arterioscler Thromb Vasc Biol 2003;23:365–7.

[7] Burman K, Ousman Y, Devdhar M. Chapter 12 – Endocrine Function in Obesity. In: Edocrine Education. 2009.

[12] WHO. Obesity: preventing and managing the global epidemic. Report of a WHO consultation. World Health Organ Tech Rep Ser 2000;894:i–xii, 1–253.

[14] Krauss RM, Winston M, Fletcher BJ, et al. Obesity: Impact on Cardiovascular Disease. Circulation 1998;98:1472–6.

[15] Wilson PWF, D'Agostino RB, Sullivan L, et al. Overweight and obesity as determinants of cardiovascular risk: the Framingham experience. Arch Intern Med 2002;162:1867–72.

[22] Sowers JR. Obesity as a cardiovascular risk factor. Am J Med 2003;115:37–41.

[24] Scheinfeld NS. Obesity and dermatology. Clin Dermatol 2004;22:303–9.

[28] Calle EE, Kaaks R. Overweight, obesity and cancer: epidemiological evidence and proposed mechanisms. Nat Rev Cancer 2004;4:579–91.

[42] Eckel RH, Grundy SM, Zimmet PZ. The metabolic syndrome. Lancet 2005;365:1415–28.

[43] Bray GA. Medical consequences of obesity. J Clin Endocrinol Metab 2004;89:2583–9.

[45] Bray GA, Ryan DH. Overweight and the Metabolic Syndrome: From Bench To Bedside. Springer; 2006.

[46] Alberti KGMM, Zimmet P, Shaw J. Metabolic syndrome – a new world-wide definition. A Consensus Statement from the International Diabetes Federation. Diabet Med 2006;23:469–80.

[48] Eslick GD. Gastrointestinal symptoms and obesity: a meta-analysis. Obes Rev 2012;13:469–79.

[55] Delgado-Aros S, Locke 3rd GR, Camilleri M, et al. Obesity is associated with increased risk of gastrointestinal symptoms: a population-based study. Am J Gastroenterol 2004;99:1801–6.

[57] Nilsson M, Lagergren J. The relation between body mass and gastro-oesophageal reflux. Best Pract Res Clin Gastroenterol 2004;18:1117–23.

[61] Vincent HK, Heywood K, Connelly J, et al. Obesity and weight loss in the treatment and prevention of osteoarthritis. PM R 2012;4:S59–67.

[70] Sowers MR, Karvonen-Gutierrez CA. The evolving role of obesity in knee osteoarthritis. Curr Opin Rheumatol 2010;22:533–7.

[76] Holick MF. Vitamin D, deficiency. N Engl J Med 2007;357:266–81.

[82] Koenig SM. Pulmonary complications of obesity. Am J Med Sci 2001;321:249–79.

[83] Murugan AT, Sharma G. Obesity and respiratory diseases. Chron Respir Dis 2008;5:233–42.

[91] Beuther DA, Sutherland ER. Overweight, obesity, and incident asthma: a meta-analysis of prospective epidemiologic studies. Am J Respir Crit Care Med 2007;175:661–6.

[92] Weiss ST, Shore S. Obesity and asthma: directions for research. Am J Respir Crit Care Med 2004;169:963–8.

[99] Linné Y. Effects of obesity on women's reproduction and complications during pregnancy. Obes Rev 2004;5:137–43.

[111] Loret de Mola JR. Obesity and its relationship to infertility in men and women. Obstet Gynecol Clin North Am 2009;36:333–46, ix.

[117] Ramlau-Hansen CH, Thulstrup AM, Nohr EA, et al. Subfecundity in overweight and obese couples. Hum Reprod 2007;22:1634–7.

[133] Smith GCS, Shah I, Pell JP, et al. Maternal Obesity in Early Pregnancy and Risk of Spontaneous and Elective Preterm Deliveries: A Retrospective Cohort Study. Am J Public Health 2007;97:157–62.

[135] Cedergren MI. Maternal morbid obesity and the risk of adverse pregnancy outcome. Obstet Gynecol 2004;103:219–24.

[146] Giovannucci E, Rimm EB, Chute CG, et al. Obesity and benign prostatic hyperplasia. Am J Epidemiol 1994;140:989–1002.

[149] Taylor EN, Stampfer MJ, Curhan GC. Obesity, weight gain, and the risk of kidney stones. JAMA 2005;293:455–62.

[151] Wang Y, Chen X, Song Y, et al. Association between obesity and kidney disease: A systematic review and meta-analysis. Kidney Int 2008;73:19–33.

[163] Whitmer RA. Obesity in middle age and future risk of dementia: a 27 year longitudinal population based study. BMJ 2005;330:1360–2.

[169] Hahler B. An overview of dermatological conditions commonly associated with the obese patient. Ostomy Wound Manage 2006;52:34–6, 38, 40 passim.

[172] Razak F, Anand SS, Shannon H, et al. Defining Obesity Cut Points in a Multiethnic Population. Circulation 2007;115:2111–8.

[180] Viner RM, Haines MM, Taylor SJC, et al. Body mass, weight control behaviours, weight perception and emotional well being in a multiethnic sample of early adolescents. Int J Obes 2006;30:1514–21.

[181] Gavin AR, Rue T, Takeuchi D. Racial/ethnic differences in the association between obesity and major depressive disorder: findings from the Comprehensive Psychiatric Epidemiology Surveys. Public Health Rep 2010;125:698–708.

[186] Dietz WH. Health consequences of obesity in youth: childhood predictors of adult disease. Pediatrics 1998;101:518–25.

[190] Lee JM, Appugliese D, Kaciroti N, et al. Weight Status in Young Girls and the Onset of Puberty. Pediatrics 2007;119:e624–30.

[195] Prospective Studies Collaboration. Body-mass index and cause-specific mortality in 900 000 adults: collaborative analyses of 57 prospective studies. Lancet 2009;373:1083–96.

[199] McPherson K, Marsh T, Brown M. Tackling Obesities: Future Choices – Modelling Future Trends in Obesity & Their Impact on Health. 2nd ed London: Government Office for Science; 2007.

## Chapter 4

[1] WHO. Obesity: preventing and managing the global epidemic. Report of a WHO consultation. World Health Organ Tech Rep Ser 2000;894:i–xii, 1–253.

[2] Butland B, Jebb S, Kopelman P, et al. Tackling obesities: future choices – project report. 2nd ed. London: Foresight Programme of the Government Office for Science; 2007.

[4] Sassi F. Obesity and the Economics of Prevention: Fit Not Fat. OECD Publishing; 2010.

[5] Swinburn BA, Sacks G, Hall KD, et al. The global obesity pandemic: shaped by global drivers and local environments. Lancet 2011;378:804–14.

[7] Pereira MA, Ludwig DS. Dietary fiber and body-weight regulation. Observations and mechanisms. Pediatr Clin North Am 2001;48:969–80.

[10] WHO. The Challenge of obesity in the WHO European Region and the strategies for response. Denmark: WHO Regional Office for Europe; 2007.

[25] Fox KR, Hillsdon M. Physical activity and obesity. Obes Rev 2007;8:115–21.

[26] Wareham N. Physical activity and obesity prevention. Obes Rev 2007;8:109–14.

[28] Bloom S. Hormonal regulation of appetite. Obes Rev 2007;8:63–5.

[30] Rolls ET. Understanding the mechanisms of food intake and obesity. Obes Rev 2007;8(Suppl. 1):67–72.

[34] Spiegelman BM, Flier JS. Obesity and the regulation of energy balance. Cell 2001;104:531–43.

[37] Diaz EO, Prentice AM, Goldberg GR, et al. Metabolic response to experimental overfeeding in lean and overweight healthy volunteers. Am J Clin Nutr 1992;56:641–55.

[38] Klein S, Goran M. Energy metabolism in response to overfeeding in young adult men. Metab Clin Exp 1993;42:1201–5.

[46] Ballor DL, Katch VL, Becque MD, et al. Resistance weight training during caloric restriction enhances lean body weight maintenance. Am J Clin Nutr 1988;47:19–25.

[48] Westerterp KR, Meijer GA, Schoffelen P, et al. Body mass, body composition and sleeping metabolic rate before, during and after endurance training. Eur J Appl Physiol Occup Physiol 1994;69:203–8.

[59] Lovejoy JC, Sainsbury A. Sex differences in obesity and the regulation of energy homeostasis. Obes Rev 2009;10:154–67.

[72] Bogen DL, Hanusa BH, Whitaker RC. The effect of breast-feeding with and without formula use on the risk of obesity at 4 years of age. Obes Res 2004;12:1527–35.

[86] Lederman SA. The effect of pregnancy weight gain on later obesity. Obstet Gynecol 1993;82:148–55.

[87] Gunderson EP, Abrams B. Epidemiology of gestational weight gain and body weight changes after pregnancy. Epidemiol Rev 2000;22:261–74.

[102] Power C, Parsons T. Nutritional and other influences in childhood as predictors of adult obesity. Proc Nutr Soc 2000;59:267–72.

[109] Finkelstein EA, Ruhm CJ, Kosa KM et al. Economic causes and consequences of obesity. Annu Rev Public Health 2005;26:239–57.

[119] Long J, Hylton K, Spracklen K, et al. Systematic review of the literature on black and minority ethnic communities in sport and physical recreation. Leeds: Carneige Institute; 2009.

[128] Lawrence JM, Devlin E, Macaskill S, et al. Factors that affect the food choices made by girls and young women, from minority ethnic groups, living in the UK. J Hum Nutr Diet 2007;20:311–9.

[147] Maio GR, Manstead ASR, Verplanken B, et al. Lifestyle Change. Evidence Review. London: Foresight Programme of the Government Office for Science; 2007b.

[148] Bell DW, Esses VM. Ambivalence and Response Amplification: A Motivational Perspective. Pers Soc Psychol Bull 2002;28:1143–52.

[151] Brug J. Determinants of healthy eating: motivation, abilities and environmental opportunities. Fam Pract 2008;25(Suppl. 1):i50–5.

[169] Froom P, Melamed S, Benbassat J. Smoking cessation and weight gain. J Fam Pract 1998;46:460–4.

[188] Nicklas TA, Baranowski T, Baranowski JC, et al. Family and child-care provider influences on preschool children's fruit, juice, and vegetable consumption. Nutr Rev 2001;59:224–35.

[196] Christakis NA, Fowler JH. The spread of obesity in a large social network over 32 years. N Engl J Med 2007;357:370–9.

[200] Roberts SB, Mayer J. Holiday weight gain: fact or fiction? Nutr Rev 2000;58:378–9.

[201] Yanovski JA, Yanovski SZ, Sovik KN, et al. A prospective study of holiday weight gain. N Engl J Med 2000;342:861–7.

[206] Lobstein T, Leach J. International Comparisons of Obesity Trends, Determinants and Responses. Evidence Review. London: Foresight Programme of the Government Office for Science; 2007.

[211] Davis A, Fergusson M, Valsecchi C. Linked Crises on the Road to Obesity: Assessing and Explaining the Contribution of Increased Car Travel to UK Obesity and Climate Crises. London: Institute for European Environmental Policy; 2007.

[216] Plantinga AJ, Bernell S. The Association Between Urban Sprawl and Obesity: Is It a Two-Way Street? Journal of Regional Science 2007;47:857–79.

[220] Giles-Corti B, Donovan RJ. Relative influences of individual, social environmental, and physical environmental correlates of walking. Am J Pub Health 2003;93:1583–9.

[223] Morland K, Wing S, Diez Roux A. The contextual effect of the local food environment on residents' diets: The Atherosclerosis Risk in Communities Study. Am J Pub Health 2002;92:1761–7.

[225] Cheadle A, Psaty BM, Curry S, et al. Community-level comparisons between the grocery store environment and individual dietary practices. Prev Med 1991;20:250–61.

[234] Li F, Harmer PA, Cardinal BJ, et al. Built Environment, Adiposity, and Physical Activity in Adults Aged 50–75. Am J Prev Med 2008;35:38–46.

[236] Mujahid MS, Roux AVD, Shen M, et al. Relation between Neighborhood Environments and Obesity in the Multi-Ethnic Study of Atherosclerosis. Am J Epidemiol 2008;167:1349–57.

[256] Cutler DM, Glaeser EL, Shapiro J. Why have Americans become more obese? National Bureau of Economic Research; 2003.

## Chapter 5

[2] NHMRC. Clinical practice guidelines for the management of overweight and obesity in adults. National Health & Medical Research Council; 2003a.

[3] Butland B, Jebb S, Kopelman P, et al. Tackling obesities: future choices – project report. 2nd ed. London: Foresight Programme of the Government Office for Science; 2007.

[5] NIH. Clinical guidelines on the identification, evaluation, and treatment of overweight and obesity in adults: the evidence report. National Institutes of Health, National Heart, Lung, and Blood Institute; 1998.

[7] NICE. Obesity: Guidance on the prevention, identification, assessment and management of overweight and obesity in adults and children (CG 43). (Guidance/Clinical Guidelines). London: National Institute for Health and Clinical Excellence; 2006.

[8] WHO. The Challenge of obesity in the WHO European Region and the strategies for response. Denmark: WHO Regional Office for Europe; 2007.

[9] Ockene IS, Hebert JR, Ockene JK, et al. Effect of training and a structured office practice on physician-delivered nutrition counseling: the Worcester-Area Trial for Counseling in Hyperlipidemia (WATCH). Am J Prev Med 1996;12:252–8.

[10] Hebert JR, Ebbeling CB, Ockene IS, et al. A dietitian-delivered group nutrition program leads to reductions in dietary fat, serum cholesterol, and body weight: the Worcester Area Trial for Counseling in Hyperlipidemia (WATCH). J Am Diet Assoc 1999;99:544–52.

[11] Pritchard DA, Hyndman J, Taba F. Nutritional counselling in general practice: a cost effective analysis. J Epidemiol Community Health 1999;53:311–6.

[17] Babor TF, McRee BG, Kassebaum PA, et al. Screening, Brief Intervention, and Referral to Treatment (SBIRT): toward a public health approach to the management of substance abuse. Subst Abus 2007;28:7–30.

[18] Artinian NT, Fletcher GF, Mozaffarian D, et al. Interventions to promote physical activity and dietary lifestyle changes for cardiovascular risk factor reduction in adults: a scientific statement from the American Heart Association. Circulation 2010;122:406–41.

[20] NOO. Brief interventions for weight management. Oxford: National Obesity Observatory; 2011b.

[21] NHMRC. Clinical Practice Guidelines for the Management of Overweight and Obesity in Children and Adolescents. National Health & Medical Research Council; 2003b.

[25] Cupples ME, McKnight A. Randomised controlled trial of health promotion in general practice for patients at high cardiovascular risk. BMJ 1994;309:993–6.

[26] Wadden TA, Foster GD, Letizia KA. One-year behavioral treatment of obesity: comparison of moderate and severe caloric restriction and the effects of weight maintenance therapy. J Consult Clin Psychol 1994;62:165–71.

[27] Steptoe A, Doherty S, Rink E, et al. Behavioural counselling in general practice for the promotion of healthy behaviour among adults at increased risk of coronary heart disease: randomised trial. BMJ 1999;319:943–8.

[28] Thorogood M, Hillsdon M, Summerbell C. Cardiovascular disorders. Changing behaviour. Clin Evid 2002:37–59.

[34] Rubak S, Sandbaek A, Lauritzen T, et al. Motivational interviewing: a systematic review and meta-analysis. Br J Gen Pract 2005;55:305–12.

[43] Pollak KI, Alexander SC, Coffman CJ, et al. Physician communication techniques and weight loss in adults: Project CHAT. Am J Prev Med 2010;39:321–8.

[48] Davidson MH, Hauptman J, DiGirolamo M, et al. Weight control and risk factor reduction in obese subjects treated for 2 years with orlistat: a randomized controlled trial. JAMA 1999;281: 235–42.

[50] Toubro S, Astrup A. Randomised comparison of diets for maintaining obese subjects' weight after major weight loss: ad lib, low fat, high carbohydrate diet v fixed energy intake. BMJ 1997;314:29–34.

[83] Knittle JL, Timmers K, Ginsberg-Fellner F, et al. The growth of adipose tissue in children and adolescents. Cross-sectional and longitudinal studies of adipose cell number and size. J Clin Invest 1979;63:239–46.

[86] National Task Force. Long-term pharmacotherapy in the management of obesity. National Task Force on the Prevention and Treatment of Obesity. JAMA 1996;276:1907–15.

[97] FDA. Drug Safety and Availability – FDA Drug Safety Communication: FDA Recommends Against the Continued Use of Meridia (sibutramine) [WWW Document]. URL http://www.fda.gov/Drugs/DrugSafety/ucm228746.htm; 2010 [accessed 21.09.12].

[103] Drew BS, Dixon AF, Dixon JB. Obesity management: update on orlistat. Vasc Health Risk Manag 2007;3:817–21.

[115] FDA. Press Announcements – FDA approves weight-management drug Qsymia [WWW Document]. URL http://www.fda.gov/NewsEvents/Newsroom/PressAnnouncements/ucm312468.htm; 2012a [accessed 21.09.12].

[117] Flum DR, Belle SH, King WC, et al. Perioperative safety in the longitudinal assessment of bariatric surgery. N Engl J Med 2009;361:445–54.

[122] Dixon JB, Straznicky NE, Lambert EA, et al. Surgical approaches to the treatment of obesity. Nature Reviews Gastroenterology and Hepatology 2011;8:429–37.

[123] Smith BR, Schauer P, Nguyen NT. Surgical Approaches to the Treatment of Obesity: Bariatric Surgery. Med Clin North Am 2011;95:1009–30.

[129] NIH. Gastrointestinal surgery for severe obesity: National Institutes of Health Consensus Development Conference Statement. Am J Clin Nutr 1992;55:615S–619S.

## Chapter 6

[2] Cecchini M, Sassi F. Tackling obesity requires efficient government policies. Isr J Health Policy Res 2012;1:18.

[3] NICE. Obesity: Guidance on the prevention, identification, assessment and management of overweight and obesity in adults and children (CG 43). (Guidance/Clinical Guidelines). London: National Institute for Health and Clinical Excellence; 2006.

[5] Gortmaker SL, Swinburn BA, Levy D, et al. Changing the future of obesity: science, policy, and action. Lancet 2011;378:838–47.

[6] Butland B, Jebb S, Kopelman P, et al. Tackling obesities: future choices – project report. 2nd ed. London: Foresight Programme of the Government Office for Science; 2007.

[13] WHO. The Challenge of obesity in the WHO European Region and the strategies for response. Denmark: WHO Regional Office for Europe; 2007.

[14] WHO. Population Based Prevention Strategies for Childhood Obesity. Geneva: World Health Organization; 2010b.

[16] Khan LK, Sobush K, Keener D, et al. Recommended community strategies and measurements to prevent obesity in the United States. MMWR Recomm Rep 2009;58:1–26.

[17] Kumanyika S, Jeffery RW, Morabia A, et al. Obesity prevention: the case for action. Int J Obes Relat Metab Disord 2002;26:425–36.

[19] Musingarimi P. Obesity in the UK: a review and comparative analysis of policies within the devolved administrations. Health Policy 2009;91:10–6.

[21] Swinburn B, Egger G, Raza F. Dissecting obesogenic environments: the development and application of a framework for identifying and prioritizing environmental interventions for obesity. Prev Med 1999;29:563–70.

[22] Waters E, De Silva-Sanigorski A, Hall BJ, et al. Interventions for preventing obesity in children. In: The Cochrane A Collaboration, Waters E, editors. Cochrane Database of Systematic Reviews. Chichester, UK: John Wiley & Sons, Ltd; 2011.

[24] Swinburn B, Gill T, Kumanyika S. Obesity prevention: a proposed framework for translating evidence into action. Obes Rev 2005;6:23–33.

[29] WHO. Obesity and overweight. Geneva: World Health Organization; 2006a.

[30] WHO. Comparative analysis of nutrition policies in the WHO European Region. World Health Organization Regional Office for Europe; 2006c.

[31] Lang T, Rayner G. Overcoming policy cacophony on obesity: an ecological public health framework for policymakers. Obes Rev 2007;8:165–81.

[33] Allender S, Gleeson E, Crammond B, et al. Policy change to create supportive

environments for physical activity and healthy eating: which options are the most realistic for local government? Health Promot Int 2012;27:261–74.

[34] Sassi F. Obesity and the Economics of Prevention: Fit Not Fat. OECD Publishing; 2010.

[43] Eisenberg MJ, Atallah R, Grandi SM, et al. Legislative approaches to tackling the obesity epidemic. CMAJ 2011;183:1496–500.

[45] Nestle M, Jacobson MF. Halting the obesity epidemic: a public health policy approach. Public Health Rep 2000;115:12–24.

[47] Lau DCW, Douketis JD, Morrison KM, et al. 2006 Canadian clinical practice guidelines on the management and prevention of obesity in adults and children [summary]. CMAJ 2007;176:S1–13.

[49] Gostin LO. Law as a tool to facilitate healthier lifestyles and prevent obesity. JAMA 2007;297:87–90.

[51] Mitchell C, Cowburn G, Foster C. Assessing the options for local government to use legal approaches to combat obesity in the UK: putting theory into practice. Obes Rev 2011;12:660–7.

[55] Ashe M, Feldstein LM, Graff S, et al. Local venues for change: legal strategies for healthy environments. J Law Med Ethics 2007;35:138–47.

[57] Farley TA. The role of government in preventing excess calorie consumption: the example of New York City. JAMA 2012;308:1093–4.

[73] Borys J-M, Le Bodo Y, Jebb SA, et al. EPODE approach for childhood obesity prevention: methods, progress and international development. Obes Rev 2012;13:299–315.

# Index

Note: Page numbers followed by *b* indicate boxes, *f* indicate figures, and *t* indicate tables.